RUNNING FROM INJURY

Why run

And how to stop it

PETER FRANCIS

©GOAT Books

Praise for Running from Injury...

[insert your praise here]

RUNNING FROM INJURY

Copyright © 2021 by Peter Francis

Edited by

Cathal Dennehy

Cover & illustrations by

Dominika Stoppa

Media and marketing by

Aisling Golden & Megan Finlay

<u>Dedication</u>

For Runners Everywhere

Don't give up

Foreword

This book is about dealing with the greatest heartache any runner can experience, injury. You will gain knowledge and training methods that will help you to manage current injuries and avoid future injury. After all, every athlete wants to be able to train free from injury and achieve a consistency that allows them to improve.

The knowledge imparted in this book is presented in the form of an adventure. Peter, an everyday dedicated runner, was pursuing his dream of trying to be the best he could be. He set attainable goals and dedicated himself to fitting his life around his training. But like so many athletes, his dream was shattered time and time again by injury of one type or another. By the time Peter was pursuing his PhD in sports science, he still harbored hope of achieving his running dreams. He stepped back and took a real hard look at his running and all the associated injury problems. At first, he made a modest plan to improve the situation in the hope that it would allow him to achieve some form of consistency. The more consistent he became, the more the buzz and joy of running returned to him and the more his performances improved. In the end, Peter achieved far more than he could have dreamt of as an athlete but more importantly, he retired on his own terms and not because of injury. He still runs for fun now.

As a reader, you will receive insight into the disappointment associated with shattered dreams; but you will also receive a roadmap out of the despair associated with injury. This roadmap is in the form of an alternate training method that enables athletes to train consistently. These methods are not the conventional methods used by many long-distance runners. Great detail is given in relation to how and why these methods proved effective.

There is nothing magical about 100-120 miles per week of running. And although high-volume running methods suited me in my own running career, I found out as a coach they are not suited to many runners. I have since used many of these methods to coach runners of all levels. Athletes, of all levels, are always looking for ways to improve via new training methods. To me, the definition of education is an open mind. Read this book, you will enjoy it and come away more educated.

Gerry

About the author of the foreword: *Gerry Deegan was a world cross country silver medallist as part of the Irish team. He was Peter's first running coach at the age of 15 and they went onto to become lifelong friends. They still walk, talk, and share ideas every week.*

Contents

Section 1

Why do runners get injured

1.

I took my first step as a runner in the autumn of 2002 at the age of 15. I wore my soccer gear and a pair of flat, thin-soled Umbro shoes that would be considered fashionable trainers rather than running shoes. The first training week I would record in a diary was in September of the following year. It was a week comprising of 37-miles with a note after Sunday's 7-mile run to say "absolutely in bits after". By December of that year, I had hit 60 miles in a week and by January 2004, two months before my 17th birthday, I ran 70-miles in a week. By this point, I had shed my soccer gear and traded in my fashion shoes for a pair of 'high-performance' running shoes that were highly cushioned and had structured arch support. I managed to run 70-miles in a week again in February, August, October, and I once hit 77-miles in November. During the year I ran personal bests over 1500m, 3000m, 5 miles, 10km and I managed a top-20 finish in the national cross country. Barely a year old as a runner, I had made rapid progress in a short time. But two weeks after my 77-mile week, I developed flu-like symptoms which began a series of viruses and infections that lingered for several months. Injury would follow my return from illness and try as I might, I would never run 70-miles in a week again. I would not run a personal best until some 12-years later. In essence, November 2004 was the beginning of a journey that would eventually lead to this book.

Too Much of a Good Thing

Many of today's chronic diseases are thought to be contributed to by recent and rapid changes in our physical and nutritional environment. Type 2 diabetes, once considered a rare disease confined to adults, is now rife in adults and has begun to emerge in children in the last 20 to 30 years.[1] There are no known archaeological records of brittle bone disease (osteoporosis) in our ancestors but now it is one of the major causes of fractures.[2] Type 2 diabetes is contributed to by high energy availability combined with low levels of physical activity and osteoporosis is contributed to by insufficient stress to bones pre and post skeletal development and insufficient high-quality nutrients.[3,4]

These diseases are described as mismatch diseases. To better understand a mismatch disease, we need to take a look at human history. The human body evolved slowly over the course of millions of years to be adept at hunting and gathering.[5] In this context, farming may be considered a very recent development at about ~10,000 years ago. Farming allowed humans to settle due to an ability to stabilise and increase food supply. The physical activity required to farm remained similar to that of our hunter gatherer ancestors. The industrial revolution which occurred a little more than 200 years ago facilitated mass production of energy-dense and sometimes nutrient-deficient food at a fraction of the human labour cost. Since then, and with the assistance of technology, our daily lives have become increasingly sedentary and our food increasingly processed. Viewed in this context, time frames we might consider large are actually minuscule in terms of the evolution of the human body.[2] It is not hard to see how our modern lifestyles are a shock to the human body and how mismatch diseases develop. Of course, access to a sustainable food supply and the elimination of excessive and potentially dangerous labour are a triumph of our time, but it is clear that too much of a good thing is bad for us.

A running injury occurs when there is a mismatch between the loading applied and the physical preparedness (also influenced by psychological readiness, see chapter 7) of your musculoskeletal system. Many coaches and runners are sometimes surprised when I suggest that injury, very simply, occurs due to a training error. The most common running injuries occur due to gradual overload. Although it is difficult to be specific, this process usually takes somewhere between a week and up to a few months. We are largely unaware that an injury is developing until we first experience pain. For example, the total running mileage of club runners in one month is not linked to running injury in the same month, but is significantly associated with the number of days injured the following month.[6] There are similarities with our modern mismatch diseases in that respect. It takes years of poor lifestyle in order to receive a diagnosis of diabetes. Although the disease process of diabetes is on-going, we are unaware until we develop symptoms.

Understanding Load

Runners would be forgiven for assuming that reference to load simply refers to miles or kilometres run. To better understand load and how it influences our injury risk, it is necessary to use some everyday examples. Have you ever gone for a run, played a game of football (soccer) or participated in group exercise after a long break? If you have, I am almost certain you will have felt very sore the next day. Have you ever bought a new pair of shoes and experienced discomfort as you got used to them? If you are a runner, have you ever run in an unfamiliar environment like a soft sandy beach, a forest trail or an unusually hilly environment and the next day, feel muscles you didn't know you had? These are your body's natural responses to novel changes in the environment. The soreness you experience the next day could be considered a short-term mismatch between the loading we experience and the physical readiness of our bodies. If you continue to expose your body to the same loading at an appropriate dose you will find that your body adapts and you no longer feel sore. Conversely, if you continue to expose yourself to the same loading at an inappropriate dose, you will develop an overuse injury. Therefore, sudden changes in running load, shoe type or training routine can influence injury risk. It is not the activity or the shoe per se, rather the change in loading.

Understanding Physical Readiness

Have you ever wondered how our bridges and buildings seldom fail despite being subject to such high loads? Our modern-day bridges and buildings are physically ready for the loading placed upon them because the material they are made of is fixed and predictable. Based on the laws of physics and the materials used, it is relatively straightforward to calculate the material and architecture required to tolerate the maximum loading (plus a safety net for some more). Our physical readiness is a lot more variable and influenced by several other factors including our genes, environment, age and current fitness level.

I mentioned at the beginning of this chapter that our bodies had evolved over millions of years to be active hunter gatherers. Given that our modern environments emerged relatively recently, our bodies are still very much designed for this purpose which includes an ability to walk and run long distances. Running is essentially a hopping action that requires us to spring from one leg to the other while not losing our balance and being able to maintain a steady gaze. Over the course of millions of years, we evolved a spring-like arch in our feet, a long Achilles tendon and large gluteal (bum) muscles to facilitate this running action. The arch and Achilles help to store and release energy and the large gluteal muscles provide the stability between the trunk (torso) and lower limb that help us to avoid falling over.[5]

How might our modern environment influence our physical readiness for running? Just like a lack of physical stress causes our muscles to shrink and our body fat to increase, the use of modern footwear including cushioned heels and arch support removes the stress from our feet and causes them to become weak. This is compounded by long hours in which we are seated (school, driving, work and home) which reduces demand on our gluteal muscles (and many other postural muscles). Runners of my parents' generation would have reached adulthood prior to the invention of the first mass-market running shoe (~1970). It is likely that they ran with considerably less cushioning than is used nowadays. I am also confident that my parents would have spent less time seated and would have expended more energy on basic tasks such as cleaning and meal preparation. Although I was a teenager prior to receiving my first mobile phone and had an active youth, largely outdoors in the countryside, I'm sure my parents' generation were more active and that I was more active than today's teenagers.[7] These recent and rapid changes in our footwear and lifestyle habits may lead to us being less capable runners relative to previous generations. The role of footwear in running injury will be discussed at length in Chapter 6. Despite modern lifestyles potentially compromising some of the physical attributes that made us natural runners, humans are defined by their capacity to adapt and we can run on a variety of surfaces and in a variety of different shoes given time to adapt. Our modern physical conditioning may mean that the time required is a lot longer than it once was.

14

These evolutionary factors aside, predicting our physical readiness is a challenge. Our muscles, tendons and skeleton change as we develop, as we age and as we engage in physical work or exercise throughout our lives. The adaptable nature of the human body means it can vary in its physical readiness not just from year to year but from week to week. Our physiology is also strongly influenced by the psychological stress we are under which can have inadvertent effects on our body. To understand why we are prone to prescribing inappropriate and injury-inducing loads relative to our physical readiness, we must understand the decision maker.

Understanding the Decision Maker

Let's say our buildings and bridges are designed by engineers. We trust these engineers are rational in their approach. They won't sanction entry to the building or declare the bridge open until it can withstand the appropriate load. However, it is not so much a case that engineers are more rational than the rest of us (although some would suggest they are!), it is that they are dealing with objects, not themselves or other people. If there is an emotional need to satisfy, it is the knowledge that they have contributed to a fully functioning building or bridge. This would also be important to the engineer because the consequence of mistakes could range from costing the firm financially, a loss of personal livelihood (in the event of dismissal) or a worst-case scenario, loss of lives. It is sensible for the engineer to take the necessary time to ensure appropriate functionality rather than risk a disaster associated with a quick finish. Let us contrast this to the human runner making decisions for themselves.

Why do you run? There are a multitude of rational answers to this question but fundamentally humans engage in voluntary behaviours because of how it makes them feel. Whether you are an endorphin chaser, you hate running but like the feeling of fitness, you want to run a personal best or you've been an athlete your whole life and it gives you a sense of who you are – running satisfies an emotional need. Our evolutionary history has given us a propensity toward instant gratification when it comes to satisfying our emotional needs. Have you ever eaten something because you were hungry but later regretted it? Sent an email because you were angry that you wish you hadn't? Bought something you didn't really have the money for? Or perhaps, run more than you know you should or run on a day when you know you shouldn't.

My questions to you highlights our struggle to appraise short-term needs in light of long-term consequences. Perhaps the simplest data-driven explanation of this is that most of us do not save sufficient money for retirement. We are primarily concerned with now rather than later.[8] This is particularly true when the consequences of our actions are less severe, more distant and somewhat unknown. Unlike the engineer who must consider a potential risk to life as a consequence of a poorly finished bridge, the runner will at worst experience an injury at some distant and unpredictable point in the future. In other words, this week's run training takes priority regardless of the consequence it has for next week's. This is further complicated by internal (personal goals) and external (races) deadlines which tend to be fixed according to the date of the race or our self-imposed agenda (our bridge will be opened regardless of whether the materials are ready or not!).

To apply subtle running loads to a variable material (muscles, tendons, bone) requires a sophisticated decision maker and often we are far from sophisticated decision makers (See Chapter 8).

How much is too much?

To improve fitness, you must place a stress (e.g. running) on the body for it to adapt. At what point does this stress lead to injury? The short answer is when the rate of change in training stress relative to your current fitness level becomes too much. Dr. Tim Gabbett has been at the forefront of research into load management in athletes in recent years.[9] Tim identified a training threshold, above which professional rugby league players had a 50-80% greater chance of sustaining an injury. The researchers developed and used this model to predict who would become injured. They were correct in predicting a staggering 87% (121/139) of injuries that occurred. Using the information from this model, they managed to halve the number of soft-tissue non-contact injuries.

Somewhat counter-intuitively, Tim found that athletes who performed a high volume of training at an intensity that wasn't overly stressful were actually protected from injury. This type of training allows the athlete to become fitter over an extended period of time and subsequently, able to tolerate loading increases at a later date. This type of training could be interspersed with a low volume of high-intensity training without further injury risk. The most risky form of training was actually when athletes engaged in a high volume of moderate intensity training. I surmise that this is because this form of training is at a high enough intensity to stress the body but a low enough intensity to be sustained for a long period of time.

Again, counterintuitively, athletes with low training volumes and long recoveries can actually be at a higher risk of injury. This is because when an athlete with a low training volume attempts to increased loading, it represents a greater change in workload. Take athlete A, who runs on average 50 miles (80km) per week for an extended period of time (~6 weeks). This athlete can comfortably accommodate the addition of an extra 5-mile moderate-intensity run, which represents a 10% change in his loading. Then take Athlete B, who runs 25 miles per week but decides to do the extra run with athlete A. Athlete B experiences as much as a 20% change in loading. This relatively small increase in training (5 miles) has drastically different consequences for injury risk in both athletes. Dr. Gabbett reported that the rugby players who experienced changes in loading in the region of 5-10% relative to their normal training load had a <10% chance of injury. Those who experienced an increase of >15% saw their injury risk jump to 21-49%.

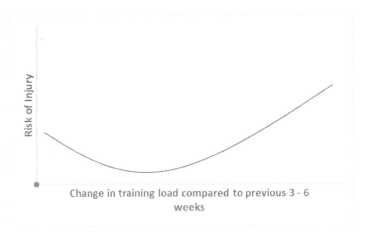

Change in training load compared to previous 3 - 6 weeks

There is evidence to support Tim's logic in runners. In runners training for a marathon, those who included tempo or interval running during the early stages (weeks 1-6) while running <40 miles per week were 4 times more likely to be injured than those who did not.[10] In other words, sudden changes in intensity without sufficient development of a higher volume of lower intensity workload (or general fitness) results in a massive injury risk. Conversely, regular participation in interval training has been found to be a protective factor against running injury.[11,12] By now you should be able to identify that it's not the 'interval training' or the 'mileage' that matter on their own, but the change in physical workload relative to the state of physical readiness.

But is there a total number of miles that increases the risk of injury?

For most of those training for distances from 10km to the marathon, a threshold of around 40 miles exists.[13,14] As you will know by now, the use of an arbitrary value to define injury risk for an individual is futile. However, this 40-mile guide may have some uses. It may be that 40 miles, the time it takes to complete (including the associated recovery), is a manageable training load for those juggling full-time employment and associated life stresses. There is no definitive evidence to suggest that this is the case but over the years with trial and error, I have come to notice this threshold more frequently in athletes I coach or during my own training. The key is to find your personal threshold, and bear in mind that it can move over time. In my own recent experience, the average number of miles I ran over an 8-week period to run 34:20 for 10km was 32, although it should be noted the overall training load was much higher when supplementary (yoga, cross-trainer, weight room) training was added. Six months later that threshold was 44 miles and in my case, I found it difficult to go much higher based on my fatigue levels. The 40-mile threshold, which should not be fixed, may be of value to the runner or runner's clinician who, when planning a training programme or taking a case history, could at least have a flag in their mind when a training plan adds up to >40 miles. The threshold will become more or less relevant when the rate of change in loading required to achieve the total is investigated.

The question the runner should be asking themselves at the end of this chapter is: are those on high mileage at greater risk of injury because of the mileage? Or is it that runners aiming for high totals, when recovered from injury, must undergo a sudden change in loading to return to a previous training status? If a runner once ran 50 miles a week, they will likely believe they should be able to repeat the feat. What the runner will tend to forget is that they didn't always run 50 miles a week and this was most likely built up to over time. During injury, our body has no reason to respond or adapt. Subsequently, our tissues detrain further and lower the load tolerance of our materials. After injury, a runner who tries to resume a training regime they were once much better adapted for is at significant risk of re-injury. It is no surprise therefore that previous injury is the biggest predictor of future injury. It is likely that regular injury and the variable loading patterns associated are highly related.

Summary

- Modern environments and lifestyles may be interfering with our capacity to be the natural athletes we once were.
- Rapid changes in loading (distance, pace, time, surface, footwear, other training) that are sustained lead to overuse injury.
- The physical readiness of an athlete is highly variable.
- Emotional decision making increases the likelihood of injury.

A training log from the winter of 2004. Training was already becoming more fragmented and punctuated by injury and illness.

2.

In the summer of 2005, I was a hungry 18-year old athlete with little interest in stopping for an autumn break, so I didn't. I began to log miles (usually 10), on most days of the week, with my coach (the author of the foreword of this book). In the middle of August, I entered an undulating 5-mile road race in which I finished 4th in a time of 26:48. For the next few weeks, I was greeted by fellow runners and former internationals from around my local area with comments like "That is some running for a guy your age". In my head, I had made it. I had trained hard and run a personal best I could be proud of. This level of training and performance was my new yard stick or reference point. For the next two summers, I entered this race usually after injury-disrupted seasons and struggled to times somewhere between 27 and 29 minutes. I was consumed by my reference point but even more so by returning to the training regime which preceded it. A glance at my training diaries reveal a consistent reduction in the peak mileage (from ~70s to 40s) reached between 2005-2013, after which I stop recording until 2016. Not only does the maximum mileage lower but the diaries become more and more fragmented by injury. There is little in the way of

consistency. Part of that was due to chasing my
reference point.

The '*Damned*' Reference Point

The personal best is perhaps the easiest reference point to recount for a runner but usually there will be a period of training preceding the personal best that the runner can clearly recall. The personal best and the training associated often become deeply intertwined in the runner's mind as a measure of success. Humans have associative brains. In other words, we are hard wired to store prominent memories which alert us to symbols of danger, safety or opportunity. The downside of this is that we store only the dominant memories and often forget the complexities associated with our experience. A good example of this might be when a football team is doing well. We naturally attribute praise to the manager. It provides us with a simple and easy-to-understand explanation of why the team is doing well. This explanation starts to fall apart when the same manager moves to a different team and does not do so well. If we reflect on our previous explanation, we realise that there are many factors that explain an outcome. In this case, the players, the fans, the chairman and the general group dynamic between those people. There are many more examples of this concept in everyday life. In the context of the runner, a good training block (the dominant memory) is used to explain the outcome (the personal best). The runner ignores complexity in two ways: 1) there was a gradual build up to the level of training undertaken and 2) the training pattern that led to the personal best in some ways is the same training that led to the injury. It is not uncommon to hear a runner say something to the tune of *'that time I ran X for 10km, I was doing Y miles per week without a problem'*.

The Insanity of Doing the Same thing & Expecting the Same Result

Initially, for a brief period after injury, a runner will be content with the simple pleasure of being able to run again. They will be in no rush to progress mileage and they will be telling themselves a story of mistakes they will avoid in future: *'I'll do my stretching this time'*. This period is short-lived and, of course, the stretching was most likely not the problem. After brief respite, the runner will attempt to aggressively pursue the reference point. In order to get to the training load that preceded their personal best, a dramatic rise in training volume is usually required. Unlike when they first became a runner and slowly moved from nothing to something, the runner will be less patient, progress too quickly and as we have seen in chapter 1, eventually pay the price. It is perhaps unsurprising that previous injury is the most significant predictor of future injury.[14] It would be easy to assume that this is because previously damaged tissue doesn't recover fully but it is highly likely that the repeated sudden changes in training load in pursuit of a former self plays a strong role (in addition to alterations in neuromuscular control and psychological state; see Chapter 7).

Unfortunately, most runners will go through many more injuries before making this connection. The reference point is magnetic. Consequently, runners attempt to travel the same path using similar training principles and inevitably end up with similar results. The definition of insanity is doing the same thing and expecting different results. Although the runner is beginning to lose their sanity, they are not expecting different results; they are expecting the same result they got the first time – *the reference point*. The reference point for the injured runner is largely unhelpful as it delays them engaging in the process that will be required to achieve consistency and subsequently performance improvement.

Reference Points: Old and New

Eventually, after enough injuries and if the runner still has the desire to return, they consider alternative training approaches to what they have used in the past. However, in the early stages of this process, the inability to fully let go of the reference point often leads to a hybrid approach. New ideas are incorporated into the training regimen with plenty of the old. In my experience, the runner often attempts to maintain the majority of the previous training load, sacrificing only a small piece they deem to be least important. The result is often an increase in training load rather than a modification. Consider the runner that runs 10 kilometres on Monday but has recently discovered strength and conditioning training is important to reduce injury risk. Potentially that runner now runs 10 kilometres in the morning and completes strength and conditioning training in the evening. The difficulty for the runner in the early stages of this process is that they haven't been able to assess the bigger picture. They don't connect that being tired for strength and conditioning negates the associated benefits. A successful strength programme often requires the mastering of technique and the ability to work muscles close to their force-generating capacity. The average runner who has never trained twice a day before will inevitably arrive to strength training fatigued and compound this fatigue by adding further training load. That damned *reference point* just won't go away.

In many respects, this was my own journey from old reference points to new. By 2009 I had a sports science degree and had begun to coach athletes successfully. By 2014, I had a physical therapy degree and a PhD. Despite this, it was not until 2016 that I began to make progress in my own running. I had to be able to integrate the sum of my experiences and education in a way that reflected the bigger picture and prioritised consistency. Doing this allowed me to generate a completely new reference point free from previous reference points in relation to myself and others (See Part 2). For a long time, I used a variety of hybrid approaches. All of them brought about some short-term success but inevitably all of them failed due to a lack of understanding of the underlying principles. To use our example above, you might know that strength and conditioning is important but understanding how to do it, why you're doing it and where it fits into the bigger picture, takes a bit longer.

The Price of Comparison

We came to a sudden halt, hunched over and gasped for air. Subsequently, my training partner and I had to walk the remaining 2 kilometres of our 'long run' back to our house. I remember as soon as I stopped running feeling as though every muscle in my body was rapidly seizing up. It is a story my friend (James) and I still laugh about now when we look back. We had decided to do a 13-mile long run with two international runners, Tom and Liam, who had recently moved into our housing estate. We had declined their offers of group training runs for a few weeks while we attempted to improve our fitness but eventually, they insisted we join them for their 'easiest' run. James and I knew within 4-miles it was not an 'easy' pace for us and ceased to waste any oxygen on conversation after that point. Both unwilling to sacrifice our pride, we doggedly kept pace with Tom and Liam while they spoke to us with ease. Eventually, I had the brain wave at a natural turn off point to announce that James and I would need to turn off as we were only down to do 10-miles that day. We bid farewell enthusiastically, as if we had been out for a stroll, made sure we were out of sight and hunched over to gasp for air. The price of comparison for us was a few days feeling more than a little sore.

The reference points of previous training load and personal bests are at least confined to the individual and could be considered internal reference points. In many aspects of our life, we are also subject to external reference points or social norms. We tend to compare ourselves to others as another strategy to assess how well we are fitting in with social norms. In the case of a runner, the external reference point refers to other runners and the training other runners are doing. A 2011 study in the *Clinical Journal of Sport Medicine* revealed that although female marathoners who trained in a group were more satisfied with the training process, they were also nearly 2.5 times more likely to be injured.[15] Trying to keep up with or match the training efforts of others is another example of how reference points can be most unhelpful.

The Long Game is Too Long

Our preference for short termism blinds us to the fact that the volume of training repeated over weeks and months will have a far greater influence on our fitness when compared to achieving a magic number (70 miles in my case) in the short term.

To illustrate this concept, let us use runner A and B from the previous chapter. Runner A can run 60 miles per week for 10 weeks before an injury occurs (a total of 600 miles). If we accept that performance is largely determined by the volume of training[16] undertaken, 600 miles will lead to a certain level of performance. Now let us consider runner B. Runner B can run 40 miles per week but can do it for 20 weeks without an injury. Runner A has completed 600 miles and runner B has completed 800 miles. Furthermore, while runner A has better early training statistics, they cannot compete due to injury and cannot improve further due to a break in training. Runner B has accomplished a greater overall training load, can race but also has the opportunity to improve further with subtle increments in training. On returning from injury, runner A remembers the elation associated with running their personal best but is quick to forget that 60 miles per week will require a substantial rise in training volume at a risk of further injury.

Runners are subject to two main reference points: 1) their previous best (race or training) effort and 2) what other runners are doing. These reference points are compounded by an assumption that more is better. From an early age we are taught that more education is better, more exercise is better, cleaning your teeth more often is better etc. In fact there is lots of evidence to suggest that the more practiced individuals are in any skill, the better they perform.[17] Runners capable of greater practise (training loads) perform better. The trouble is that when we are injured, *we can no longer practise*.

Summary

- As soon as a runner completes a run of any distance, they have a reference point.
- A reference point usually refers to a runner's best performance.
- The runner's best performance is usually achieved after a period of training. This means the source of the

runner's best performance is often related to the source of the injury.

- Runners struggle to let go of the methods that led to their reference point which often impedes a return to consistent running.
- Runners intuitively will favour a short-term, high-volume training load over a long-term performance gain.

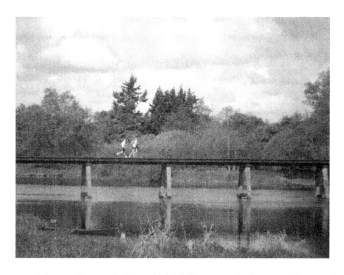

From a distance: *James (left) and I (right) eventually became fit enough to run with Liam (centre) for a while at least. Photo taken by Patricia Barry on the banks of the River Shannon, Limerick, Ireland.*

3.

My retirement from running was first suggested by a physiotherapist when I was 19. I was attending for persistent hamstring tendon pain. This was the beginning of a belief which suggested that when it came to being able to run, I was fundamentally flawed or as coaches might remark, 'very injury prone'. At that time (2006), the average athlete was at the mercy of what they were told by a clinician. Six years later, diagnostic scanning was a lot more common. These were the scan results I received for persistent heel pain in 2012: **There is marked thickening of the plantar fascia. This measures over 8mm in thickness (normal is less than 4mm). A 1.2cm tear is noted and there is also calcaneal (heel) bone marrow oedema**. The findings were upsetting to say the least. I didn't know it at the time, but my brain would interpret my distress as a threat and in order to protect me, made sure the pain sensitivity in my heel remained elevated for some considerable time afterwards. As the injuries, clinicians and diagnostics mounted over the years, the story about the fragile nature of my body became entrenched. It would be some years later before I knew how to re-write the script because once you know what is 'wrong' with you, it can be very hard to go back.

It is only a small stretch to say that recovery from the most common running injuries is made more difficult by a clinician. This may sound counterintuitive considering that most clinicians genuinely aim to help you. However, the way in which clinicians have been trained means they are prone to focus on two things which are often (not always) unhelpful: a) the diagnosis and b) the cause or reason for that diagnosis. An injured runner usually presents with pain but can leave a clinician's office with pain, a diagnosis and a cause. The diagnosis and the cause serve as the explanation for the pain. Together, these three things form a story. We are storytelling creatures and find comfort in being able to explain why the world around us is the way it is. Stories help us reduce and cope with the uncertainty in our world. Stories can make us feel sad (bad news, uncertainty) or happy (good news, safety) depending on how our brain perceives the story. Perception is why two people can experience different reactions to the same story. Many of the stories we tell ourselves and each other are inaccurate or at best overly simplistic. This is certainly the case with running injury.

Any diagnosis implies that something is different to normal which in our primitive minds is at least threatening. The cause or reason for the diagnosis may be more or less threatening depending on the extent to which we believe we can rectify the situation. If the cause we are presented with is poor shoes we may feel it is easily fixed but if it is perceived as irreparable (e.g. a structural 'fault' in our skeleton) we may become more anxious. Lastly, the experience of pain has been hardwired for millennia to represent bad news (often with good reason). All in all, these three items (pain-diagnosis-cause) that make up our story are a potent mix of threat and uncertainty. In the case of a runner, running becomes a threatening activity that may lead to further damage. The natural response of the brain is to protect against further damage by keeping pain signals elevated (more on this in Chapter 7). The runner now starts to develop a fear of the activity which led to the pain and underestimate their body's ability to cope. This becomes heightened as the number of injuries increase. Pain, diagnosis and cause are the foundation of a story that depicts our bodies as fragile and unable to cope. Unfortunately, this story is very often untrue, but our brain doesn't know that.

Diagnosis: Fact or Fiction

Runners will be aware of terms such as 'leg length discrepancy', 'fluid around the knee', 'a thickened Achilles'. These terms are often received after a trip to an expensive medical professional and, increasingly, with the addition of even more expensive imaging technology. In reality, many runners will have 'abnormal' findings and be completely pain free. Research demonstrates that swelling, particularly in the foot and ankle, comes and goes naturally even in professional runners.[18] Signs of damage in the knee joint as measured by MRI are no different in marathon runners compared with those only recreationally active[19] and Achilles tendon thickness is not associated with symptoms of pain in club runners.[20] Even in healthy runners, the presence of fluid around the outer knee is subject to dramatic variability depending on the angle of the knee during assessment.[21] Perhaps more telling is that in older adults, with a confirmed diagnosis of knee osteoarthritis, those with the highest pain sensitivity had the lowest radiographic evidence of damage in the knee.[22] This study teaches us that pain and symptoms associated with injury are not necessarily associated with structural changes evident on scans.

The Uncertain Cause of an Uncertain Diagnosis

By this point, we have presented with a pain, let's say in our knee. We have had an assessment or a scan and received a diagnosis. At this point, we crave an explanation. The reality of the explanation is likely very grey. Even at the early stage of this book we know that some form of training or loading error (Chapter 1) has occurred and that there may be psychological drivers such as 'reference points' (Chapter 2) playing a role. That is before we even discuss the many other factors at play. Yet, the clinician is prone to offering us a rather specific factor, usually about our body, for us to fixate on as the reason for our diagnosis. Weak hips, the wrong shoes, flat feet and training on tarmacadam are a selection of the causes we might be offered. Some of these factors or a combination of some of these factors may play some role in our experience of pain but it is likely a small one and it is definitely overly simplistic to explain the complexities of pain in this way. For example, screening of lower-limb characteristics such as hip angle, leg length and ankle or foot position have been shown not to be linked to injury in runners who were measured and followed for 3 months.[23] The problem with such explanations is not primarily with their inaccuracy but the role they play in our story and our brain's perception of that story. Let's use the following story to draw these concepts together:

*'I have a **degenerative** Achilles (diagnosis). It'll never go away (permanent). I'll probably **never** run as fast again (threatening internal story). I think it happened because I have **weak** gluteal muscles on my left side (cause). I can't seem to make it as strong as the right, so it's not looking good (inability to solve problem, an internal story of a fragile body)'*

What is the cause of my injury?

As discussed above, the cause of running injury is multifactorial and the subject of the entire first half of this book. However, the level of dysfunction a person experiences from a chronic pain condition (i.e. the most common running injuries) is more closely associated with our perception of the situation and our behaviour as a result of the pain than the anatomical location. Positive outcomes in relation to pain from research studies are best predicted by changes in psychological distress, reductions in fear associated with activities and increased confidence in our ability to manage pain.[24] In spite of this, assessment and treatment of running injury remains largely focused on the anatomical structure and unsurprisingly, the prevalence and incidence of running injury remains largely unchanged[25] despite advances in 'specialised' diagnostics and treatments.

Why does the diagnosis-cause model of injury management persist?

The desire for more rather than less diagnostics is perhaps psychological and social. Psychological distress is influenced by loss, threat and uncertainty among other things. An injury threatens the athlete's ability to run and increases the probability of losing out on pre-determined goals such as a race. In other words, an injury represents an uncertain future. Humans have a deep aversion for uncertainty[8], something that is inherent with injury and something which makes diagnosis and explanation so appealing. We are willing to pay a high price for certainty. This is perhaps most simply illustrated by our willingness to have outstanding credit card debt and savings at the same time. Financially, it is better to clear the debt but we prefer the certainty of our savings. A diagnosis, particularly one with a clear explanation (cause i.e. structural abnormality) is seen as the first step to reducing the threat of uncertainty about our running future. Diagnostics provide us with an illusion of control.

It is worth remembering that clinicians are human too and they also have a need for certainty. The certainty a clinician requires is a little different to the injured runner. Imagine you attend a car mechanic with some engine trouble. Now imagine the car mechanic can't figure out what is wrong. You might not be very impressed with his mechanical skills and he might not feel great about himself given that his identity depends on the certainty he offers in being able to diagnose and correct your engine trouble. Let's just say that, not wanting to look foolish, the mechanic provides you with an explanation that he thinks might be right and says he can fix it. In that moment, you are both pleased. By offering certainty he fulfils the expectations you have of him and he has of himself as a mechanic. You are also happy about the certainty that your car can be fixed. In this hypothetical scenario, unsure about the exact cause, the mechanic adjusts as many factors as he can in the engine in the hope of a successful outcome. This is often the dance between the clinician and the runner. The runner wants certainty and the clinician is expected to have it. Another example in the field of musculoskeletal conditions is the use of surgery. In some conditions, there is mounting evidence that the outcomes are not better after surgery than they are after physiotherapy.[26] Logic would suggest, that this form of surgery would no longer persist. I suggest **part** of the reason it does is due to the surgeon's need for certainty about their own identity; if a surgeon no longer does surgery – who are they?

The social aspect of our drive for diagnosis is linked to the psychological aspect. If society accepts this model of recovery, we tend not to question it. If everybody else is doing that, why should we engage in the complexities of considering an alternative path? Furthermore, clinics offering a simple and precise explanation for our woes are attractive for a runner suffering loss and desperate to avoid the threat posed by uncertainty. We are willing to pay a high price for a very uncertain 'certainty'.

Where to from here?

Polarising the argument for or against orthopaedic assessment or diagnostic imaging serves little purpose and in many instances these tools are most useful. The identification of a stress fracture is an obvious choice of injury whereby this mode of investigation is most effective. Thickening of the Achilles and patella tendon identified via ultrasound imaging are predictive of the development of tendinopathy in the future. In fact, those with thickened tendons have a four-fold greater risk of developing tendinopathy than those without thickening.[27] Whilst this information is potentially useful for the development of injury-prevention strategies, it still does not alter how we might manage the runner who actually has the condition. In this case, the thickened tendon is somewhat irrelevant; the pain and associated loss of function is what needs to be addressed; the tendon may remain visibly unchanged.

There are two key considerations in relation to the level of diagnosis and structural causes that should be offered to the patient. The first is whether the level (and cost) of investigation is 'fit for purpose' and the second is the communication of perceived 'findings'. Part of the reason I write this book is that as an athlete, I have had many of the injuries (often more than once) and treated many of them as a clinician. The most common running injuries occur from the knee down and are as a result of overuse. Although there is some variance in the literature, consistently reported are iliotibial band (IT band) syndrome, patellofemoral pain syndrome (runner's knee), medial tibial stress syndrome (shin splints), Achilles tendinopathy and plantar fasciitis (heel pain).[25,28-30] These conditions are not life-threatening, rarely require imaging and most experienced musculoskeletal clinicians (particularly those experienced in working with runners) will tell you are very manageable. Despite this, in recent years, I have noticed a worrying trend toward the pursuit of complex assessment and treatment for musculoskeletal tissue overload. I have been involved in sports science and medicine support to international athletes for 10 years now. Regularly, athletes attend clinic with diagnostic imaging reports and details of their previous injections for conditions such as IT band syndrome and shin splints. Sadly, many of these runners have not even reached 20 years of age. Some of these athletes have pursued these options having been unsatisfied with the outcomes of primary care, but others have gone directly towards these investigations believing that a more precise diagnosis will lead to a better outcome. The evidence does not support this reasoning. It is beyond the scope of this book to fully explore the standard of musculoskeletal care available to the active population and the referral pathways that lead to more complex investigations. While more complex investigations are sometimes warranted; they are a necessity if private providers are to make a profit and as a result, they will no doubt continue to find ways to prosper.

A note from before you knew what was wrong with you

The title of this chapter serves as the perfect opportunity to take you back to a time before you knew what an MRI machine or leg length discrepancy was. Imagine primitive humans roaming the earth in search of food and shelter. What do you think their reaction would be to a sore Achilles? It is hard to imagine exactly, but without knowledge of diagnosis and depending on the severity of injury and/or how hungry they were; they would either keep going at a reduced pace or take a rest along the journey until the pain subsided. Of course, should a hungry lion appear, they would still be able to sprint away or climb a tree. In other words, the pain is not life-threatening. Do you think they would reflect upon the thickness of their tendon or the length of their legs and the role it might have played? I doubt it. Were they better off without this knowledge? Possibly, if not probably. Of course, whether the pain had fully subsided or not, at some point they would need to continue their journey. In other words, there would be some level of load maintained through the tissue at all times. Rest would serve little purpose in the completion of the journey or in the long-term health of his tendon.

In Conclusion

Regardless of the findings obtained via manual or imaging assessments, of greater consequence is the delivery of information to the patient. As discussed above; thickenings, fluid build-up and anatomical discrepancies are present in many athletes who are completely pain free. Such findings may or may not be related to the experience of pain for an injured runner. However, to the emotionally compromised runner, the perception of a 'serious' injury can have devastating consequence for the rehabilitation process and their long-term perception of their body (discussed in chapter 9). There is a growing body of evidence which suggests that chronic pain (the pain most common to runners) is influenced by biological, psychological and social factors.[31,32] The role of psychological and social factors in pain perception will be discussed in chapter 7. The purpose of their mention in this chapter is to suggest that great care should be taken when considering an assessment fit for purpose and in the subsequent communication of the relevant findings. Clinicians needs to realise that: *once you know what is 'wrong' with you, it can be very hard to go back.*

Summary

- Diagnosis seen on imaging can also be present in runners with no pain and in healthy adults who do not run.
- The label of a diagnosis can sometimes do more harm than good especially if it is accompanied by a cause that will only be partly related to the problem, if at all.
- Diagnosis and cause can be used to provide an explanation for pain. This often creates a story which depicts a runner's body as fragile or in some way flawed. These stories are often highly inaccurate and always overly simplistic.

- The experience of pain is often more to do with our perception of the situation (story) and our ability to rectify or manage the situation than it is with the anatomical site.

Findings:
There is marked diffuse thickening of the calcaneal insertion of the medial bundle of the plantar fascia, this measures over 8 mm in thickness (normal less than 4 mm).
The involved fascia is diffusely heterogeneous, with interstitial 1.2 cm long tear noted.
Bone marrow oedema is present within the adjacent calcaneum.
No fascial retraction seen.

An MRI report I received in 2012.

4.

The first running injury I ever had was commonly known as shin splints. I remember my shin bone being exquisitely painful to touch. I went on to have others such as hamstring and Achilles tendon pain, IT band (outer knee) pain and plantar fasciitis (heel pain, 3-times). I began to notice these injuries had something in common. They came on gradually and in the early stages, a warm-up was enough to eliminate the pain. As they got worse, they became painful to touch in a specific area and they almost never involved my muscles. In 2008, I met a physical therapist (John Stacey) who helped me to make progress with several recurring injuries. My rehabilitation and conditioning strategy always seemed to awaken muscles I didn't know I had. It seemed training which involved muscular soreness was key to reducing the strain on what seemed to be non-muscular injuries. Some years after my first visit to John, I was conducting research into sports injuries; I noticed that sprinters and professional footballers mainly suffered from muscle injuries. I began to wonder, what is it about the way sprinters and footballers behave that means they use their muscles a lot more and very rarely suffer from these slow developing, long-lasting and very painful conditions that are present in distance runners?

With every foot-strike, the runner must absorb collision forces with the ground. The musculoskeletal system is primarily responsible for for absorption of these forces. The stress placed on this system needs to be balanced and proportionate. For example, we would expect muscles to produce and absorb more force than ligaments, because that is a muscle's primary function. Running injury occurs when one aspect of our musculoskeletal system is stressed disproportionately relative to its intended purpose. The best way to illustrate this concept is with an experiment. With hands on hips, jump as high as you can and land by bending your legs to cushion your impact. Next, jump as high as you can but land with your legs fully extended. I do this experiment with different audiences by taking a selection of the crowd and getting one group to land softly and the other to leave their legs extended. I then ask the rest of the audience and the groups themselves to comment on the difference. These are the answers they usually come up with:

Jump 1 (Soft)	Jump 2 (Hard)
Quiet	Loud
Soft	Hard
Gradual	Sudden
Comfortable	Painful
Smooth	Vibration

The next challenge I set the audience is to explain to me, using their intuition, why there is a difference between both landings. After all, the jump height, their body weight and gravity haven't changed so why would there be such a difference in the experience of landing? The difference of course is in the parts of the musculoskeletal system being used to absorb the forces. Jump 1 makes use of a number of large muscles on the front and back of the body to cushion the landing. Jump 2, relies largely on the skeletal system (e.g. bones, joints, ligaments, plantar fascia) and the quadricep muscles which work to provide stability at the knee and maintain knee extension. The skeletal system is not designed to absorb such large forces.

Muscles, in addition to absorbing force, are designed to produce force. Asking those performing jump 1, to jump a second time after landing is straight-forward. In a crouched position, their joints are flexed allowing muscles to forcefully extend the limbs so that the person becomes airborne again. For those performing jump 2, immediately jumping a second time is impossible as they are stood with legs extended in an upright position.

Now that you understand the difference between using the musculoskeletal system in balanced and unbalanced ways to absorb force, how does this translate into running and running injury? The image below illustrates what it is like to run using the hard landing strategies of the jumpers in group 2.

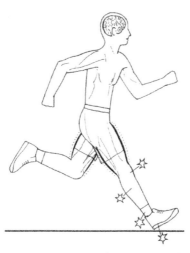

Just like the jumpers in group 2, the runner is landing with legs extended. The stars represent the most common running injury sites (knee, shin, achilles, plantar fascia). Notice, none of them are to muscular tissues.[25]

The Long-Term Effects of not using Muscles

Muscles adhere to the principle of 'use it or lose it'.[33] Imagine you took part in a circuit training class and when you reached the squat jump station you jumped like instructed in jump 2 (legs straight). Apart from the fact that landing would be uncomfortable, the main muscle you would use is the quadriceps. This would allow many muscles such as those around your hips and on the backs of your legs to essentially fall asleep. The largest muscle that seems to suffer as a result of these jumping (or running) mechanics is the gluteal muscle complex, otherwise known as your bum. This muscle was arguably the most important in our evolutionary development from primates who were on all fours to being humans on two legs.[34] This did not happen overnight and the transition to being the superb long-distance walkers and runners that we are (should be) would have taken some time. Nonetheless, a key change that facilitated this was the pelvis turning sideways (rather than backward in primates) and large gluteal muscles being able to anchor our torso to our lower limbs so that with each step we would not fall over. This is important, as running is essentially a series of hopping actions from one leg to the other and falling over might have meant death. The image below illustrates what happens when our gluteal muscles become weak or fatigued during running.

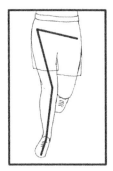

The consequence of gluteal muscle dysfunction is that the knee begins to collapse inwards and there is increased stress along the inside of the knee and shin bone. There is also a tendency for the foot to roll inwards (pronation). These mechanics have been linked to a number of running injuries.[35] It appears that there are direct consequences (stress to the musculoskeletal system) for using upright and extended mechanics during running but also longer-term consequences for the muscles not being used when running in this way.

How does the sprinter or the footballer avoid the runner's injuries?

Although running is the main protagonist for injury in sprinters and distance runners, that is where injury similarities end.[36] The initial clues for why this is are in the image below.

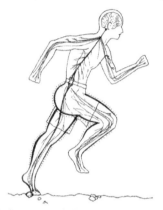

The sprinters left leg is in full extension about to make the athlete airborne. The right leg is bent. It will begin to straighten before foot contact, but never fully so that it can act as a spring to absorb some of the collision forces before straightening the leg again to return to the air (much like jump 1). You can observe this in real-time by watching a YouTube video of any 100-m race. In essence, the sprinters run in such a way that muscles always have mechanical advantage, this is necessary for speed but it is also why other parts of the musculoskeletal system are rarely overloaded. High forces, at high speed, as muscles lengthen under tension (known as an eccentric muscle contraction) is likely the main reason that sprinters injure their muscles in a way that distance runners do not.

Unlike sprinters, footballers do have to run around for 90 minutes. Therefore, it might be expected that they would experience more injuries like the distance runner. The reason this is not the case, I suspect, are two-fold. Firstly, football is a repeated sprint activity and therefore likely uses the muscle-dependent mechanics of the sprinter. Secondly, footballers are required to run at a variety of speeds as well as change direction, throw, jump, kick and head the football. Therefore, the major advantage the footballer may have over both the sprinter and the distance runner is variability. The requirement for greater movement variability will likely use the musculoskeletal system in a variety of different ways.[37]

The primary reason for the mention of footballers in this chapter is to highlight two major challenges faced by the distance runner: 1) insufficient use of muscles to control repetitive landing and 2) a lack of movement variability. In part two of this book, we will address the issues that make us more susceptible to overloading our skeletal system. How can we behave more like a sprinter but at lower running speeds? How can we have the variability of a footballer, but without the football? How can we develop landing mechanics like jump 1 rather than jump 2? Finding the right answers to these questions may well unlock the secret to a lifetime of happy, healthy running.

Summary

- Collision forces with the ground need to be absorbed by our musculoskeletal system in a way that is balanced and proportionate so that no single tissue is overloaded.
- Running injury is mainly to skeletal or non-contractile tissue and rarely to muscle. This suggests these tissues are being overloaded during distance running.
- Running mechanics that allow the legs to act like springs are required to reduce the impact of collision forces.
- Sprinters and footballers appear to use mechanics which load (sometimes overload) muscle and this appears to spare them from the injuries experienced by the distance runner.

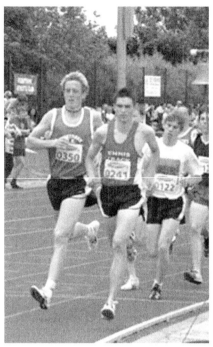

My running mechanics (runner 0350) were not helping me in 2005.

5.

*It was December 2017, and I had been running for two years consistently. I had just completed a physically and mentally demanding block of training in preparation for a race, which was ultimately cancelled due to snow. My body and mind were tired and Christmas was approaching. I granted myself some rest in the form of two easy weeks. In week 1, I did 3 runs and none of the usual supplementary training (yoga, strength & conditioning). In week 2, I did 2 runs and had 4 straight days of complete rest. My mind enjoyed the break and the festivities. The persistent pain in my right Achilles tendon, which I had for the previous 4 years, also began to settle down. January began in earnest with a swift return to my pre-Christmas routine. I did not foresee a problem; after all, it had only been a short rest period. My Achilles tendon thought otherwise and the pain soon began to soar to unprecedented levels. In this instance, **rest** had signalled the beginning of the end of my consistent streak. I would be forced to stop running not long afterwards.*

Doing too little can be just as dangerous as doing too much when it comes to the risk of running injury. Studies on astronauts or patients confined to bed rest demonstrate the severe consequences associated with a lack of mechanical stress on our musculoskeletal system. The loss of muscle mass, bone mineral density and tendon stiffness, in as little as 7 days, are startling.[38,39] Most runners do not experience this level of extreme rest but equally, most runners are a lot more active than the average person. If a runner ceases to run, it represents a dramatic unloading of their musculoskeletal system compared to their normal levels. This means that returning to running represents a significant rise in loading. If the rest period has been long enough, it may mean loading tissues that are ill-prepared to cope. In essence, this is how rest feeds into the message of Chapter 1. The diagram below illustrates the negative rest cycle.

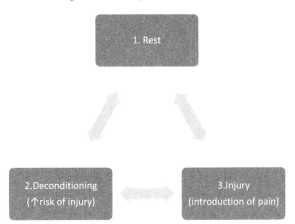

Rest vs. Recovery

Rest may be viewed as a blunt instrument for a complex problem. Recovery is its more sophisticated sibling. The everyday example below illustrates how rest and recovery are integrated for optimum results. We will then consider where I went wrong with my rest strategy in December 2017.

Example: Think of a time you were gripping something you normally do not, like the handle of a shovel or the handle of the rowing machine at the gym. Later that day you develop callouses on your hands because you are not used to it. As a result, you will avoid the **specific** activity for a day or two (rest) until the pain goes away. But while you avoid that specific activity, you do not stop using your hands; in other words, your hands do not decondition. Your hands recover rather than rest.

Where did I go wrong in December 2017?

It may have appeared as though there was a large drop in my running, but the reality is, I was only running four days a week to begin with. I ran three days during the first easy week and despite four days off, I still ran two days the following week. The real issue was dropping from seven days, during which my tendon was always loaded, down to two. Training loads in my pre-Christmas schedule included resistance exercise, yoga, plyometric training and circuit training – in other words, anything but rest. This was added to by my everyday loading such as my 20-minute walk to work and the significant number of hours standing and walking while delivering lectures and teaching practical classes. To provide a direct comparison to our analogy above, even on the days I was not running (resting the callouses on my hand) I was still exercising the tendon (using my hands).

Although, that is where I erred in my recovery strategy, there were other forces at play, some of which we have already discussed in this book. In January, I was chasing my pre-Christmas reference point (Chapter 2) and this required a significant increase in training loads (Chapter 1), alongside a return to my everyday loads. The sensible strategy would have been to accept that I had had a significant rest period and gradually rebuild my training load like any pre-season period. Psychologically this proved difficult for me due an internal reference point (my pre-Christmas training) and an external reference point (a race in March).

Conclusion

There is an obvious danger in writing a chapter that may be understood as anti-rest, whereby athletes confuse the concepts of rest and recovery. Recovery is essential to improved performance and reducing injury risk. Rest may be viewed as a blunt instrument for a complex problem. Recovery is its more sophisticated sibling. It is for these reasons that the traditional advice for musculoskeletal injuries, which composed of the acronym RICE (Rest, Ice, Compression and Elevation) has recently been replaced by POLICE (Protection, *__Optimal Loading__*, Ice, Compression and Elevation).[40] As we will see in part 2, a consistent, moderate load is key for tissue health and performance. Even for the injured runner, we will examine how you can remove the aggressor (running) and still load the injured tissue. We will also discuss how you can rest multiple energy systems and musculoskeletal tissues in the same week by varying the training applied to healthy and/or injured tissue.

Summary

- Rest is a blunt form of recovery, useful in certain situations but sometimes detrimental when applied for lengthy periods.

- Musculoskeletal tissue health declines rapidly without mechanical stress.

- The resumption of training after rest periods ≥7-days requires a sudden rise in training volume and therefore, carries an increased risk of injury.

25 Monday

9:00 am

10:00

11:00

Noon

1:00

2:00

3:00

4:00

5:00 pm

26 Tuesday

9:00 am

10:00

11:00

6 miles
Cloned 4 miler race

Noon

1:00

2:00

5:23 pace

3:00

21:24.

4:00

5:00 pm

27 Wednesday

8:00 am

10:00

11:00

Noon

1:00

2:00

3:00

4:00

5:00 pm

SIGNATURE PARENT ☐ YES

13

Thursday 28

9:00 am

10:00

11:00

Noon

1:00

2:00

3:00

4:00

5:00 pm

Friday 29

9:00 am

10:00

11:00

Noon

1:00

2:00

3:00

4:00

5:00 pm

Saturday 30

7 miles

Sunday 31

20 x 60 sec
(30 sec rest)

SIGNATURE TEACHER ☐ YES ☐ NO

Running 2 days out of 7, was a significant reduction in my normal load.

6.

Once I became a serious runner in 2003, I always had serious shoes. Variants of structured, semi-structured, arch supported or neutral shoes but always highly cushioned and usually highly expensive. There is only one thing that can make a running shoe more expensive and that is the orthotic you put in it. This was particularly true in my case when I booked a flight to Belgium for a custom fitted pair of orthotics in late 2011. The process involved running up and down a track (barefoot and in a variety of shoes at different speeds) while being videoed and having pressure plate measurements taken. It is ironic now to look back at the videos to notice that the pronounced pronation in my right foot was all but gone when I ran barefoot. Had I understood what I was observing at the time, I might have saved my money and gone barefoot or at least held onto my original flat-soled Umbro shoes. Six years later, when I embarked on an almost uninterrupted 3 years of consistent running, there was lots of barefoot training and the shoes I did use for training or to run my fastest ever times were light, comfortable and very cheap.

I began to write this book in 2017. The World Championships were on in London that year and I came across an interview with a member of the refugee team. Below is an extract which perhaps best highlights the scale of misunderstanding when it comes to running shoes.

He is one of the lucky few there to have proper training shoes, which he feels is essential for athletes to continue chasing their sporting dreams. "Most of the time it was difficult to train," he admits. "We didn't have the right shoes and trained in the wrong ones and got injured. Now, some have them, some don't, so I hope people can hear our stories and support the people there." Gai Nyang – interviewed by Cathal Dennehy, 22nd April 2017.

Gai Nyang is an 800m runner who trains in the Kenyan hills where running or walking barefoot is as natural to people as water is to a stream. It is testament to the power of marketing emerging from industrialised countries, that it can convince Gai Nyang that something he and his ancestors have evolved to do over many millennia contributes to running injury. Put simply, there is no evidence that shoes reduce the likelihood of running injury, but most runners still believe it to be true.

A brief history of shoes

Humans have walked and run barefoot for millions of years.[41] Indirect evidence suggests that footwear emerged as recently as ~30,000 years ago.[42] The majority of time since then, humans have worn minimalist footwear designed to protect the sole of the foot.[43] The first indication of fashionable footwear beginning to alter the shape of the foot emerged a

60

little over 100 years ago[44] and the invention of the mass-market cushioned running shoe is as recent as ~1970.[45] Therefore, large changes in footwear have occurred in a very short space of time relative to human evolutionary history. As discussed in Chapter 1, rapid changes in our environment have a propensity to drive mismatch disease. Differences in foot structure between those who have never worn shoes and those who are habitually shod have been described since 1905.[44,46-49] Although the study is over 100 years old, Hoffman, in describing the absence of weakness-associated symptoms in 186 pairs of 'primitive feet', warns that the characterisation of the foot as 'vulgar and unsightly' is in favour of the 'dictum of fashion' and the 'manufacturer's self-interest' rather than 'reason'.[44] Fashion was also suggested as the primary reason for an increasing number of African adults wearing shoes in spite of poor fit. The purpose of the shoes was not for protection or utility but rather to mimic the white man and demonstrate superiority to their peers.[46]

The first mass-market 'cushioned' running shoe was not manufactured until some 70 years after Hoffman's initial warnings about the use of everyday footwear. It was of great surprise during the research for this book to discover an unsubstantiated narrative about the benefit of running shoes toward the aim of injury prevention in the scientific literature. In the 1980s, 'better running shoes' were suggested as a reason for the reduced incidence of Achilles tendinopathy in one study and 'poor shoes' suggested as a risk factor for stress fractures in another study.[50,51] In the early 1990s one intervention study used 'proper individually fitted running shoes' and did not allow for light competition shoes.[52] Yet, in 2009, a systematic review entitled '*Is your prescription of distance running shoes evidence-based?*' could not find a single study which met the inclusion criteria for review and was forced to conclude 'the prescription of this shoe type (cushioned heel or pronation control systems) to distance runners is not evidence-based.' A year later, a randomised controlled trial (the highest level of experimental study) investigating the effect of three different levels of footwear stability on pain outcomes in female runners concluded that shoe prescription for over-pronation was overly simplistic and potentially injurious.[53] The findings of similar studies in thousands of military personnel have drawn the same conclusion.[54,55]

How shoes change our feet

Those who grow up barefoot tend to have wide feet and a well-defined arch. Shoes do not allow the foot to splay and reduce the workload on our foot muscles, the result is a narrower foot and a collapsed or flattened arch due weakened foot muscles.[49,56,57] Shoes usually contain a heel, which holds our calf and Achilles in a shortened position. The padding in the heel and throughout the rest of the shoe dampens the information to the nerves in our feet. Over time, this means we use a more blunt walking pattern. The combination of the factors outlined above is thought to contribute to higher peak pressure at the heel and just beyond the arch in shod populations.[48,58] By contrast, habitually barefoot populations demonstrate more equally distributed peak pressures toward the outside of the foot and toes.[48,59,60] An example of what this looks like on a pressure plate measurement is provided below.

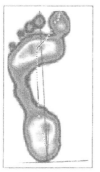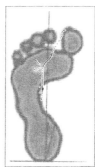

How shoes change the way we run

During barefoot walking or running, as the foot meets the ground, the skin, ligaments, tendons and nerves of the foot feed a rich source of information to the brain and spinal cord (see image below). The quality of this information allows the precise control of muscles to move our joints into a position (spring like) that absorbs impact in a way that limits damage. These innate systems that all humans possess will be discussed in part 2 of this book along with strategies for how to develop them.

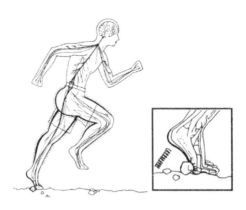

Footwear reduces the quality of information to the brain and spinal cord leading to more blunt running mechanics (see image below). Shoes allow runners to land with a more upright body position and an extended leg, leading to excessive braking forces. These running mechanics seem to play a role in some of the most common running injuries.[25] Barefoot runners appear to report less knee injuries and less heel pain (plantar fasciitis) compared to shod runners.[61] The impact of footwear on injury risk may not be limited to running mechanics. As discussed above, long term use of everyday footwear leads to a weaker foot and often, a collapsed arch. The injurious running mechanics described above are being inflicted on a foot that is not adapted to cope. If we combine the factors of a reduction in the quality of information to the brain, a reduction in foot muscle size and strength, excessive breaking forces on landing and less conditioned lower limbs (discussed in Chapter 1 and 4) it is not difficult to see why we might suffer more injuries than our hunter-gatherer ancestors.

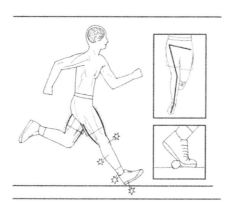

Why shoes persist

Recent scientific literature is replete with investigations that, if compiled under one umbrella, could be summarised as: 'An investigation into the effectiveness of barefoot running...'. However, as barefoot activity has been the default state for many millennia, it seems strange that investigations do not read: 'An investigation into the effectiveness of shoes...'. The development of a drug or treatment designed to enhance or assist our bodies' natural physiology always asks the question in this order. We assume the eyes can see best until we have evidence that glasses make it better, and we don't then prescribe glasses to people who can see perfectly well. We consider the effectiveness of a drug for heart disease and weigh it up against the risks to the individual. We use clinical trials to assist us in making these decisions and we have doctors who practise from a standpoint of doing no harm.

Why not apply the same logic to running shoes? We are uncertain about the long-term consequences that running shoes may have on our feet or health, but in the short term they pose no major threat. This is coupled with the fact that we need something to protect our feet from skin perforation and extreme temperatures. That something might as well be fashionable and if there is even a chance that it might reduce injury, then why not? By contrast, we know that the wrong drug can kill us and so there is greater regulation of what medical professionals are allowed to prescribe.

There are parallels between the shoe and the sugar industry. The habitual use of carbonated drinks is unlikely to alter your health now, but it might later. What protects both the shoe and the sugar industry is the absence of any major short-term consequences and the number of other attributable factors available to blame when disease occurs. For example, as changing loads and previous injury (Chapter 1) are the major players in running injury, it would be very difficult to uncover the shoes' contribution to injury. In much the same way, it would be hard to determine the contribution that regular ingestion of carbonated drinks makes to a person's diabetes some years later.

The parallels continue in the treatment of disease. Governments (unfortunately) and pharmaceutical companies (naturally) focus far more energy on the treatment of disease relative to its prevention. In our western capitalist society, this allows the generation of revenue at both ends i.e. when you buy the sugar and later, when you buy the medication. Footwear is now being developed in much the same way. Excessive pronation associated with weak ankle and intrinsic foot musculature is being counteracted by motion controlled shoes.[62]However, much like a stent in the heart, it only addresses one aspect of the problem. Part 2 of this book will discuss how a combination of being barefoot and some simple footwear criteria may assist in the prevention of injury associated with every day and athletic footwear.

What about the super-shoes?

Performance is built on a foundation of health. That is why this book focuses very much on addressing the barriers to consistent injury free running. You will see in part 2 of this book, that consistency is the dominant factor in all performance improvement (and in your everyday life). That being said, it would be remiss of me not to comment on arguably the biggest development in running shoes since their invention in the ~1970's.

The super shoes improve running economy[63] and performance.[64] Anything that reduces the mechanical work needed to be undertaken by the runner will artificially improve performance. Studies and athletes have demonstrated this.[63,64] However, in chapter 1, 4 (especially) and 5 you have learned that reducing work on muscles and tendons causes them to become weaker. In fact, it has been demonstrated that even the upward curvature of toe springs in normal athletic shoes reduces the work performed by the toes[65] and likely contributes to weakening of the foot muscles. Therefore, use of the super shoes for short term performance gain must be balanced with the same risks associated with the use of all modern cushioned footwear - deconditioned foot muscles and tendons and potentially more injurious running biomechanics.[66]

Conclusion

It should be noted that running injury is influenced by many factors which is why there are 9 other chapters in part 1 of this book. And while shoes are relatively new to our species, so are many of our modern surfaces, as are the concepts of prolonged sitting and other sedentary behaviour. It is likely that this results in humans being less conditioned for long-distance running in ways they might have been before. It will be tempting, on reading this chapter, to think that the solution is a world without shoes and certainly keeping children barefoot or in minimalist shoes seems wise, however, when it comes to the individual, an already shod runner, the solutions are rather more nuanced than that, so make sure you read part 2 of the book.

Summary

- There is no evidence that shoes (of any kind) lead to a reduction in running injury.

- Those who do not wear shoes growing up have stronger feet and a more even distribution of pressure underneath the foot.

- Shoes reduce the quality of information transmitted to the brain and spinal cord leading to more injurious running biomechanics.

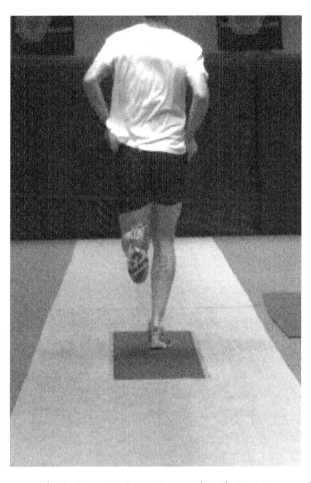

Being assessed prior to purchasing custom made orthotics in January 2012.

7.

I had conquered most of my running injuries but for the remnant of one, my Achilles heel. The pain in my right Achilles tendon hung around, reminding me of sins from my past. It didn't stop me running, usually, but intermittently it would flare up in ways that would force me to modify training for a week or two. The final piece in the jigsaw of consistent running would be getting to know and understand this pain. I spotted a trend during December 2015 (Christmas), April 2016 (a foreign training camp) and August 2016 (a foreign holiday). The trend was an increase in my run training volume and consistency (consecutive days running) without any appreciable change in my overall experience of pain. The thing that connected all 3 experiences was that they took place in novel environments and the training undertaken did not have a defined outcome (a race or training reference point). In other words, training was frequent but unstructured. Returning from my holidays, I glanced through my training diary and to my surprise; I had run almost every day for a month. I began to wonder why my pain didn't get any worse despite the increase in the volume and frequency of running. It appears the relationship between pain and function is not straightforward.

There are 3 components to my experience of pain in the above story. The first is the state of the tendon's health (biological), the second is my perception of the training load and other life stress (psychological) and the third is my location (environmental). The traditional view of pain is that it is mainly biological in nature. However, there is now strong evidence which suggests that an individual's experience of pain is governed by an interplay of all 3 factors (bio-psycho-social).[67] To understand this concept, think of the biological aspect of the pain as a car running in neutral. Sat in your car, you are aware the car is running (there is pain) but you are not distracted by it and you can still have a conversation on your handsfree (you can still run). Suddenly, you notice a car coming towards you on the wrong side of the road (environment has changed). You ascribe meaning (*danger*) to this change in environment (psychological response) and you press hard on the accelerator. The revs of the car are now very high, loud and you can no longer have a conversation (the tendon is now very painful, and you cannot run).

Let us now see how this plays out for a runner. The health of a runner's muscles, bones, tendons and ligaments represents their biology. Running itself is simply the action of putting one foot in front of the other, that is of course until the runner ascribes meaning to it. Running may represent an individual's identity ('I am a runner'), a major personal goal (a race, fitness target), a method of maintaining physical and mental health ('I need this') or a combination of all the above. In this context, pain or injury and the potential loss of running represents a major threat (psychological distress). This causes the brain to press the accelerator hard and to amplify the pain. The experience of pain can be added to by other stress in our home or working environments (further psychological distress).

In my examples from 2015-2016 above, I am no longer preparing for a race or trying to attain a certain level of fitness whilst working full-time (psychological stress) and I am no longer in the environment that has become associated with that stress. With only my biology to contend with, my pain is not so bad. Of course, I cannot go on holiday or change location every time I have pain, but I can become aware of how the meaning I ascribe to my pain or my training can heighten or lower my psychological stress. If I learn that my pain (sometimes) is not as threatening as I once thought, there is an excellent chance I will be less distressed when I experience pain. Equally, if I become more attached to the process of improvement (internal goals) rather than the target level of fitness or race (external goals, see chapter 2), I will be less distressed when there are bumps in the road.

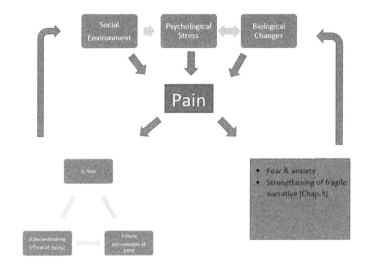

(Rest cycle from Chap.5)

When pain changes our behaviour for the better

Imagine you over-estimated your athletic capabilities and jumped from a wall that was just a fraction too high for your musculoskeletal system to cope with. As a result, you break your leg and experience a lot of pain. The x-ray of your leg confirms a broken leg i.e. why you are in so much pain. Several weeks later, the x-ray demonstrates where the leg has healed, and you are no longer in pain. You might be tempted to think, that is where the story ends, but it isn't. Your brain stores a careful record of the environment in which the event took place and the psychological distress you experienced as a result of your leap of faith. This is not so that you can tell stories of the event, it is so that the next time you find yourself on a wall, you will climb down rather than jump. In this instance, the brain has done a marvellous job. It has used pain to prevent further damage and it has also stored the memory so that you don't do it again. This is how the interaction between biology (pain), psychology (distress) and environment (a high wall) interact to help us avoid danger.

The difference between acute and chronic pain

Traumatic bone breaks belong to a group of injuries known as acute injuries. This means that they are usually of sudden onset, very painful, measurable on scans, follow a reasonably predictable recovery time and often teach us a lesson. Running injuries belong to a group of injuries known as chronic injuries. This means they are usually not easy to define; their onset is slow; their pain is less intense but longer lasting and their recovery time uncertain. For example, the average recovery time for the top 5 running injuries is at least 10 weeks but can be up to 18 months.[68]

There are several aspects of human nature, some of which we have already discussed, which automatically make chronic injuries more difficult to manage.

Level of Threat: Initially, the level of threat is low i.e. a niggle that doesn't stop us from running. As discussed in Chapter 1, humans are poor at appraising the longer-term consequences of their actions on their health. It seems, we would rather run now and be injured next week, than wait for a resolution to our niggle.

Uncertainty: Humans have an aversion to uncertainty. Chronic injuries can be hard to diagnose and recovery times are more difficult to predict. As we discussed in Chapter 3, this often leads to us pursuing complex imaging and medical intervention in a desperate grab for certainty.

Prolonged and Ever-present Pain: By the time we cease running, we have a full-blown chronic pain condition (bio-psycho-social). The pain is present in many of our activities of daily living, providing a constant reminder of our injury status.

Hyper-sensitivity to New Pain or Niggles: The often drawn out recovery process can leave a runner somewhat traumatised from the experience. If this has been added to by complex diagnosis and structural abnormalities given to the runner by clinicians in Chapter 3, the runner is now hyper aware of any pain or discomfort. This can lead to heightened psychological distress with the slightest niggle, even if it may be unnecessary (their biological tissue is fine). This facilitates more cautious and rigid running mechanics, often compounding the problem.

We learned in Chapter 3 that it is possible to have physical abnormalities evident on scans but not have pain and to have clear scans but still be in pain. From this, it is logical to suggest that the experience of pain may be more psychologically and environmentally driven in chronic injuries. To use our analogy from earlier, the foot is on the accelerator. Regardless of its origin, chronic pain eventually drives fear avoidance: not participating in an activity for fear of further damage or increasing pain. The consequence of this behaviour has been outlined in Chapter 5, rest, which promotes deconditioning of our biological tissues.

Conclusion

The understanding of pain we have accrued in this chapter should help us to explain the spontaneous improvements in my running at the beginning of this chapter. The two major changes in all three cases were the environment (social context) and the meaning attributed (psychological response) to running. In a familiar environment where I was injured, going to work and wondering when I could get back running, my pain remained elevated. In this environment, I was conscious of timelines, when I could get back running, when I could race, how I would balance it with work etc. By changing the environment to something less familiar, reducing the demands of work and letting go of potential timelines, my brain began to relax and no longer see running as a threat. The morning pain and stiffness remained and represented the biological component of the condition but without being amplified by the psychological or environmental factors, the pain intensity never reached a threshold that would interfere with running. In other words, I began to separate pain and function. I could have pain and still function. Pain did not necessarily represent excessive tissue damage, which allowed me to gain control over my pain rather than other way around. Understanding these concepts is essential to avoiding excessive rest and deconditioning but also to enhancing compliance to rehabilitation aimed at reducing pain and enhancing function.

I have illustrated the separation of pain and function with an example from when I was recovering with Achilles tendinopathy in 2018.[69] The blue line represents my pain score out of 10 (10 being very bad) over a period of 16 weeks. During the first 5 weeks, the pain score was >4 out of 10. This pain is somewhat akin to the leg break pain, in that there is a strong warning not to run. Running is re-introduced after 5 weeks, to which there is an initial surge in pain. However, from week 6 onwards, there is a continuous rise in running volume or intensity and a continued lowering of pain down to <3 out of 10. At this point, pain is not interfering with increasing function.

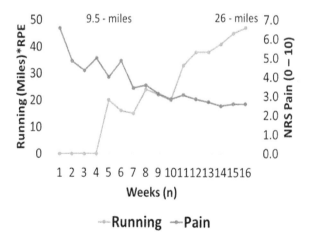

RPE = rate of perceived exertion (effort). NRS = numeric rating scale (pain score out of 10)

Summary

- Pain has biological, psychological and environmental components.

- The pain associated with biological tissue damage can be higher or lower depending on the psychological appraisal of the damage and the social context in which the runner operates.

- Pain and function are linked but not as closely as previously assumed especially in chronic pain conditions.

8.

I ran for 40 weeks uninterrupted during the 2010-2011 season, the longest streak between my first brush with injury in 2004 and eventually becoming consistent in 2016. This was partly due to discovering the benefits of barefoot running on playing fields in 2010. Very quickly, every physiological measure (heart rate, lactate threshold, body composition) and training statistic became the best I'd ever had. I competed twice for the University in 2011 (a success in itself). On the eve of a track meet in 2011, I found myself run down and dropped out of the 5,000m the following day. I carried a bug for a further two weeks. On my return, I completed a track session which involved running 800m repetitions in 2 minutes 20 seconds and 400m repetitions in 63-65 seconds. I was very fit but at the end of the session I couldn't even warm down due to the pain in my left foot. I would be out for a further 11 weeks. It may appear as though I went from making great progress to a disaster very abruptly, but to be honest, I had it coming. I was a full-time PhD student doing long hours in the laboratory every day, a weekend student studying for a BSc in Physical Therapy, the university endurance coach and I was involved in a host of other projects. As I limped off the track that day, part of me was relieved. I was mentally exhausted. My inability to delay gratification, work on a small number of projects and treat my running with the respect it deserved, meant I just didn't have the headspace to run at that level. After 40 weeks, I became very fit, sick and then injured.

In many respects, it is very easy to be an injury-prone runner. I never had to concentrate on my training for too long before the next rest period came along. Consistency requires a discipline that injured runners rarely experiencen If you train too hard, too quickly or juggle too many other balls in your life, the chances are you have a tendency toward *instant gratification.*

The Theory of Self Control

'You can have one good training session now or two good races later' – is how I imagine the runner's version of the marshmallow test would be administered. The marshmallow test is a test given to young children to test their self-control. Over many years of research, children were offered a treat, which was placed in front of them, and they were told that if they waited until the researcher returned to the room, they could have two treats. If at any time they wanted to have one treat immediately, all they had to do was ring a bell. The longer the children waited during the marshmallow test, the higher their self-control. Amazingly, performance on the test as a child was linked to success in many facets of their life as adults – psychological, emotional and social. Does this mean that if you have low self-control you are doomed? No. What the researchers also found was that by reappraising the treat as a less desirable object the children could increase their waiting time.

The origin of such behaviour comes from two different places in our brain. The impulsive part of the brain, described by Professor Daniel Kahneman as system 1[70] or the hot system,[71] and the rational part, described as system 2 or the cool system. The hot system has primitive origins and is key to survival instincts such as hunting, reproducing, escaping a lion or slamming on the brakes of a car. The cool system thinks more about future consequences – two treats will ultimately be better than one or saving for retirement now instead of buying a BMW will lead to greater satisfaction later. The hot system acts quickly and sometimes automatically, but the cool system is slower to react. Although the cool system is more rational and concerned with our future selves, it requires constant effort to be engaged. This tussle between systems is often what makes breaking a habit difficult. I can enjoy that cigarette now, but I might get lung cancer in 20 years' time. Overall, we are far more concerned with our immediate selves.

Self-Control in the Runner

To friends and family, runners are often seen as models of self-control owing to their relative fitness and dedication. For a time, I used to wear this accolade with pride, until I realised, I was more than a little ill-disciplined. Think of the satisfaction that comes from a moderate-to-hard 60-minute run. You're feeling good and swimming in a sea of endorphins on your return. Relatively speaking, you have received instant gratification for your efforts. Now think of that race that you could have performed better in, had you avoided a run like that two days beforehand, or think of that injury you picked up because you ran every day on your week off work.

At the time of your 60-minute run you could not activate the cool system 2 sufficiently to fully appraise the longer-term consequences of your instant gratification. Research suggests that had you been primed before that run you may have acted differently. For example, had someone said to you, 'would you like to run fast now or in two days at the race?' Or if someone said, 'would you like to run every day this week or four days a week for the next seven weeks?' Or, 'remember how you felt the last time you were injured?'

These leading questions are attempts to get you to activate the cool system 2 and act in a way that protects your future self. The runner with the new personal best at the race will be happier than the one who has left his best effort on a local road two days earlier. The busy office worker will be physically and mentally in a healthier place should she run for seven weeks in a row versus seven days in a row.

Headspace and Self-Control

The more you require concentration from the more rational part of your brain, the more you deplete its fuel stores. You may have heard this expressed as having less 'headspace'. This is often why individuals who start an exercise regime fail to lose weight. They have used all their head-space reserves to get the exercise done in the morning and go to work. In the evening, with their reserves of self-control used up for the day, they treat themselves to extra calories which keeps them in a state of balance. If work was particularly stressful that day, they may even over-indulge as depletion of headspace can come from many sources.

Running with a goal or reference point in mind requires headspace because it adds a layer of meaning. It is no longer about keeping fit, instead it is like solving a complex problem. In this case, running is more akin to a discipline than a sport. If a runner is depleting their head-space reserves outside of running, there is a good chance their run performance will suffer; much in the same way a muscle does without fuel. We have already seen, how psychological stress increases pain sensitivity (Chapter 7). In my story above, we see how low headspace led to underperformance, illness and injury. The sense of relief I felt was due to being able to relinquish the headspace required for demanding track sessions, it was one less job to deplete my already limited headspace. At other times, I have noticed low headspace manifest in ways that mean I am less motivated to perform the tasks necessary for injury prevention. I call them the little extras like warm-ups and cool-downs, yoga, cross-training and rehabilitation exercises. In times of low headspace, we revert to type (hot system 1) which is often repetitive running routes with little imagination in terms of pace or distance and none of the supplementary training. This can lead to injury due to not using our muscles often enough and a lack of variability as discussed in Chapter 4.

Conclusion

Our need for instant gratification combined with low headspace reserves can make us very inflexible in our thinking towards injury-free running. Unfortunately, low headspace can lead an athlete to question whether they have fallen out of love with the sport. In part 2 of this book we will discuss how we can delay gratification and learn to tolerate or even enjoy the boredom associated with doing things consistently. We will also look at strategies to increase headspace and how increased headspace allows the love of running to come back.

Summary

- Humans have a primitive urge to pursue instant gratification. This leads to us focusing on the immediate future without consideration for long term performance or injury prevention goals.

- Self-control is needed to reduce injury risk in the runner. Reduced headspace reserves limit our ability to exert self-control. If life stresses are high, it will be difficult to exert the self-control needed to reduce injury risk.

- Old habits die hard. Headspace is required to come up with creative solutions for behaviour change to avoid running injury.

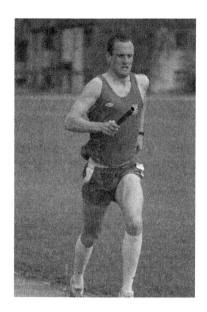

Flying fit in April 2011 at the University of Limerick, but on the verge of disaster the following month (below).

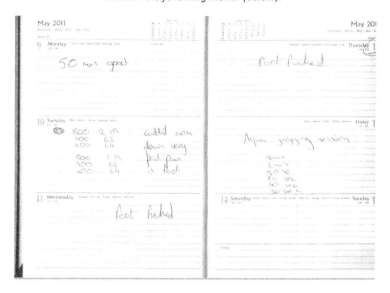

9.

I limped off the playing fields and back to my car with considerable pain in my heel. What made me stop running that day? I'm not sure. I guess it always reaches a point when you just know, the game is up. I had been using pain killers for several weeks which had slowly become less able to mask the pain, until one day it was too much. I felt the shame wash over me, as I contemplated being asked 'was I injured again?'. I was out for a good 5 months and I didn't do much to help myself. Take away for dinner and beer for the weekend. Eventually, my friend Lynne prodded me towards some open-water swimming and cycling and slowly the running came back at some point, I'm not sure exactly when.

I've lost count of the number of times over the years when I knew the game was up but couldn't accept it. Accepting it is the first step to resolution and accepting it sooner rather than later limits damage and shortens recovery time (sometimes to mere days). Viewed in this way, denial of reality serves no beneficial purpose. So why do it? In every case, it was the story I was telling myself, a story not based on reality, but a story built by the 'ego'. I was denying injury in favour of clinging to a narrative. I could not let go of my current story or plan in favour of a new modified one.

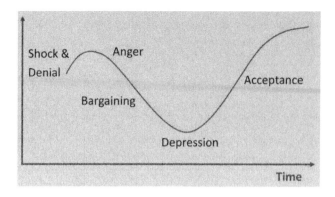

The process has been compared to grief.[72] Denial is in relation to the loss of your narrative, your story about yourself and your goals. Bargaining usually follows. In my case, I was usually only a short number of weeks from my goal, and I would start to think about how I could manage myself toward the start line with my fitness intact. This can be a successful strategy if a niggle is developing the week of a race or follows a known pattern with rest and recovery (Chapter 7). It does not work when you have been injured for some time and denying it. Sometimes, I would start to remove all but the key running sessions in favour of cross-training. This and or some medication (I never used medication until later years when I was close to giving up) would get me closer to my goal and closer to the day I had to stop running. I usually had one more bargaining tool up my sleeve in the form of a complex treatment or intervention, usually recommended to me by another junkie (I mean runner). After a brief dance with hope, it usually failed, and I was officially injured. I would promptly move into despair and begin using negative coping mechanisms such as a lack of exercise and increased junk food and alcohol consumption. Acceptance and recovery often took weeks and even months to arrive.

Despair can be the longest and has the greatest potential to harm the rehabilitation process. Limiting the length of this phase is key. If the athlete has been injured frequently, a sense of helplessness can develop. Some form of denial and bargaining is inevitable, but the sooner the athlete moves through the phases of anger and despair toward acceptance, the sooner they will be back running. Thankfully, in the later stages of my career there were fewer injuries and niggles (due to the learnings in this book) but when bumps in the road did appear, I could accept them very quickly. The despair phase became very short due to an awareness of what was happening and what needed to happen to get better. I was very quickly able to switch from injured runner to athlete in training within a week i.e. training hard without running. In other words, I could accept the end of one story and begin a new one which served me better.

Conclusion

The real problem with athletic injury is not the individual injury itself but the narrative it becomes part of in the runner's mind. In the closing words of this chapter, it is worth addressing the runner's narrative.

The runner's narrative is formed from a combination of chapter 2 (the reference point), chapter 3 (before you knew what was wrong with you), chapter 7 (no brain no pain) and this chapter (denial).

These chapters represent the set of experiences of the runner: their training, their injuries, their goals and what they have been told about them. To make sense of our lives we summarise these experiences into a story about ourselves – the narrative. The trouble is that this narrative is just a summary, think of it like a one-line description of a movie and often it is not completely accurate. This is compounded by the fact that just like any science textbook, our narratives become outdated several times in our lives but still we cling to them.

Summary

- Denial of niggles or injuries usually leads to more damage physically and mentally and prolongs recovery time.

- The use of medication or complex treatments for an injury that has been developing over time usually do not work.

- Letting go of old stories or plans and creating new modified plans reduces the severity of injury and length of recovery.

- Limiting the number of injuries and their severity is important to avoid building a fragile narrative about yourself and your athletic capabilities.

10.

Chapter 1 referred to a 12-year period of on-off injury beginning in 2004. This period was not without glimmers of hope. In 2008-2009, I ran for a 16-week and 25-week stretch having been introduced to strength and conditioning. In 2010-2011, a combination of strength & conditioning and barefoot running on grass led to a 40-week block of training. Why then did it take another 5 years before I would run for almost 3 years and break the personal bests of my youth? The answer is the difference between information and knowledge or, more colloquially, the ability to see the wood from the trees.

Pieces of *information* are like the parts of a car. They are useless without the *knowledge* of the mechanic who can put them altogether in a way that allows the car to work. The mechanic's knowledge allows him to problem solve when it is not quite right or provide a short-term fix until there is time for further repairs.

My stint in 2008-2009 was akin to the ignition making a sound and my stint in 2010-2011 was akin to the car beginning to roll in neutral. As I learned about strength and conditioning and barefoot running; I was amassing my own information via 3 science degrees and multiple coaching qualifications.

Each time I made progress with my running was the equivalent to two pieces of information being joined together to form a little bit of knowledge. But as the saying goes, 'a little bit of knowledge is a dangerous thing'. In 2008-2009, progress in my running, with overly simplistic reasoning, becomes associated with strength and conditioning. This led to me worshipping at the alter of strength and conditioning and encouraging other runners to do the same. When someone takes a singular piece of information and puts it forward as a cure all it is known as 'dogma'. Dogma is often professed by a 'guru'. A 'guru' is usually someone who has had a positive experience as a result of a singular piece of information or someone who is well educated in a narrow field and forms an identity around sharing their information with others (physiotherapists, strength & conditioning coaches and social media influencers can all be gurus). As there is usually some truth in the information, it is likely that others will have some positive experiences which creates a following. All is well until the information ceases to have the same effect (in my case being injured again) or there are enough people who don't have the same positive experience and they begin to form a dogma of their own. This can leave us in a permanent state of confusion. To observe a guru in action, sign up to Instagram or Twitter but be kind, we are all on a journey from information towards knowledge (hopefully!).

In my case, pieces of information provided glimmers of hope towards an eventual solution. It's a bit like a scientist in a laboratory who shouts 'eureka' only to be disappointed later when they realise their knowledge on the subject remains incomplete.

A little bit of knowledge is a dangerous thing

The fact that 35 - 50% of runners are injured at any one time[25] and recovery times can vary between 10 weeks on average and up to 18 months[68] is indicative of our failure (medicine, education and others) to address the problem of running injuries.

A failure to acknowledge nuance facilitates dogma in developing. A runner who attends a medical practitioner with an injury and has a successful resolution due to a specific treatment will worship at the altar of that therapist. This will then reinforce that practitioners knowledge. But there is a good chance that both parties are being fooled by randomness. In reality, the resolution of an injury will be due to a combination of:

- The passage of time
- Factors related to activities outside of treatment
- The empathy received from the therapist
- A placebo effect
- The specific treatment being appropriate for that specific injury in that particular individual.

Does it really matter provided the runner gets better? Yes. In our example, the runner develops a belief that their therapist has the solution to all injury problems. They have learned little from the experience and rather than developing skills to manage their musculoskeletal health, they view the solution to running injury as completely external to them. This does not empower the runner to understand her body or manage her training loads to avoid injury. The consequences of this type of scenario do not stop there, however. They continue when runners interact with other runners and spread overly simplistic information.

In 2008, I thought that strength and conditioning improved my running economy (energy cost to run at a given speed) and improved the tolerance of my musculoskeletal system for absorbing impact on running. I'm sure this was true in part but what I would have failed to recognise is that it also:

- Added variability to my training

- Initially reduced the time I spent running

- Increased the consistency of my running via fewer injuries

Why didn't it continue to have the same effect? I didn't yet understand that there were issues with my running mechanics (related to footwear use) which meant increases in running load would still lead to some types of injuries. I didn't understand that increasing running load on top of strength and conditioning could also increase overall fatigue and injury risk.

In 2011, barefoot running seemed to help enormously. It cured my plantar fasciitis and as I was galloping around the fields, I felt great. Afterwards, I was a lot less stiff and sore than I used to be. However, I failed to recognise that my stature, style of shod running mechanics and injury profile was ideally suited to such an intervention. It helped me to shorten my stride, receive increased proprioceptive feedback from the ground, strengthen my feet and add variability through greater movement of the foot and increased deformation of the ground. I had not factored in that wearing a cushioned shoe for the rest of my day, which held my Achilles tendon in a shortened position, would then subsequently predispose the tendon to increased loading due to the more forefoot running style required by barefoot running.[73]

Why do runners get injured?

As we conclude the final chapter in section 1, I hope you know the answer to this question (at least as well as I do) and I hope you can understand why in 2011, my knowledge was still incomplete (it still is now).

Runners get injured due to a change in loading (chapter 1, 5) that often results from an inability to delay gratification (doing too much too soon) and while chasing an internal (weight-loss goal, previous best time, former fitness level) or external (race deadline, training partners goals) reference point (chapter 2). The same set of behaviours can often lead to runners having busy lives outside of running which contribute to psychological overload (chapter 8). These psychological drivers are added to by physical ones. Running is a sport with little movement variability and modern runners often use injurious running mechanics (chapter 4) and have weak feet associated modern footwear use (chapter 6). This is added to by the fact that modern life also has significantly less movement variability than our bodies are adapted for. The result of these movement patterns is that runners often use some muscles too much and others too little meaning they end up with lots of stress through joints and tissues not as well designed for managing impact.

Runners often wait too long to accept they are injured and run through niggles (chapter 9). Denial delays the process of recovery. Once injured, runners attend clinicians. Many clinicians are prone to focus too much on the physical nature of the diagnosis and neglect the bigger picture (chapter 3). This leads to runners developing a fragile perception of their bodies i.e. they become more fearful of running and underestimate their bodies ability to cope (chapter 7). In reality, the amount of time a runner misses out on training is more closely associated with what they think about pain and how that makes them behave than the structural 'damage' offered by diagnosis.

A failure to appreciate all of the above and their combined role in contributing to injury leads to an overly simplistic explanation of injury (chapter 10).

Summary of Section 1

- Any change in load (surface, running distance, shoes, stress levels, non-running activity) can lead to an injury.

- Trying to obtain a former level of fitness or personal best (reference point) without regard for the process of gradual build up risks injury.

- Diagnosis and labels placed on your musculoskeletal system in conjunction with your previous experience of pain can lead to a false narrative about yourself and your capabilities.

- Running is a repetitive and demanding movement activity that lacks variability. This increases the risk of overload to passive tissues and underuse of certain muscles.

- Rest is a blunt instrument to use for recovery and can increase injury risk.

- Wearing traditional footwear weakens the foot. Wearing cushioned running shoes can facilitate running biomechanics associated with injury.

- The brain's perception of threat, which is often determined by the runner's environment, can increase pain sensitivity.

- Runners desire for instant gratification can increase injury risk. Low headspace can make it harder to delay gratification and therefore increase injury risk.

- Denial of a developing niggle or injury will delay a return to consistent injury-free running.

- Failure to appreciate all of the above and their combined role in contributing to injury leads to an overly simplistic explanation of injury.

Section 2

How do we stop it?

11.

What a journey it has been. Running for 140 of the last 148 weeks after almost 12 years plagued with injury. That would have seemed like a pipe dream just a few years ago. Consistency brought about performance improvements. It started with accepting I was a 36:40 10km runner in 2015, before improving in 2016 (35:18) and breaking my PB by the year's end (34:20). The dream goal of a sub-34-minute 10km came in 2017 (33:46), in front of the Sydney Harbour Bridge and in the presence of my uncle and brother. It has been a great 3 years but also a long 3 years. Physically, I am better than ever but mentally, my race is run.

The paragraph above is an extract from my retirement blog post. I had tried and failed to run under 33 minutes for 10km and I no longer had the will to sustain the regimen that made such lofty goals possible. Although there was sadness in reaching the end of the road, there was triumph in retiring on my own terms and not because of injury. This book will have been a success if it allows more runners to do similar. How did I do it? That is the question that section 2 of this book aims to address.

Before we begin, I would like to share with you the personal journey I have been on to obtain the knowledge I am sharing with you in this book. I published this article shortly after I ran what remains my personal best for 10km (33:46). Reading this will set the tone for everything you are about to read.

The Road to Redemption: 10,000 hours of practice

"When an athlete gets injured, it's akin to amputating a chair's leg and expecting it to stand. The leg which supports them, defines them, disappears" – Cathal Dennehy, Sunday Tribune, 2007.

Ironically, I had been coaching at Cathal Dennehy's parent club Emerald AC for some months when I read his award-winning piece of journalism 'Nil Desperandum'. A tale of hope at a time when I was beyond hope. Aged 20, I had known little but injury or illness for the previous two years. I had turned to coaching to fill the void that running had left behind.

I would attend coaching courses usually with a group of people twice my age. Parents, volunteers and ex-athletes largely satisfied with their athletic endeavours and trying to give something back.

'Why are you doing this?'

'I do some coaching in Limerick, it gives me something to do when I'm injured.'

'Oh, so do you run?'

'Well yeah, kind of.'

'What have you run?'

'I ran 34:40 for 10km and 26:48 for 5 miles but that was when I was 18.'

'Did you run track and cross country?'

'Yeah, I finished 6th in an all-Ireland 1500m and top-20 in a national senior schools cross country but that was when I was 17. My brother won an All-Ireland cross country as a juvenile.'

'Oh yeah, I think I remember him'.

By the age of 25, I had completed all the coaching certification available in Ireland, coached at Emerald AC for 3 seasons and I was running the endurance programme at the University of Limerick for the next 3. In 4 years of university education, I had run in a solitary 5,000m on the track, in my final year, which was preceded by 12 weeks of cross-training due to plantar fasciitis in my left foot.

By this point, my developing knowledge of injury and performance was beginning to find a limited voice in the sport. I would go on my first warm-weather training camp as sports science support for Irish U20 internationals in 2011.

Back on home soil, at a coaching course, my newly researched methods for injury prevention would be laughed out of the room, classed as 'unimportant' – 'your man in Limerick doesn't have a clue what he's doing'. I was still young and emotional about the methods that had robbed me of my running. The German guy teaching the course seemed to like what I was saying – it kept me going.

For me, there would be other comebacks. During the first year of my PhD, I managed 40 weeks of training before disaster struck. The following year, I coached 15 people from our office to run a half marathon. As they made their way around the streets of Limerick, I followed them on a bike with fluids. Afterwards, toasting their success, I could barely concentrate on their exuberant stories due to the pain in my left foot. I would need pain killers for the night out.

Bit by bit, the sport wore me down. First, I would give up all ambition of track running, perceiving it as too hard on my body. I would instead focus on road racing, before having to give up racing ambition altogether.

The famous song suggests the first cut is the deepest, but in truth the cuts only got deeper with each passing injury. I became wary of the sport. Like a lover with a commitment phobia, I began to flirt with running rather than falling in love all over again. I'd make a comeback and decide not to fully commit until I started to see some returns. I would not do the little things, I'd keep going out on a Saturday night, never fully committing so that when the next injury would inevitably result, I wouldn't be as hurt. It still hurt though. What hurt more was the gradual removal of my identity.

'Do you run?'

'Ah yeah, I just do a bit to keep fit.'

'Did you compete?'

'Yeah, but that was nearly 10 years ago now.'

I was offered a get-out-of-jail-free card in 2012 – an MRI scan. 'Calcaneal bone oedema, a 1.2cm tear in the plantar fascia'. This is great, I thought, my leg is f**ked and I have a piece of paper to prove it.

In 2014, aged 27, I had given up and was training for my first half-ironman triathlon. My cousin wanted to do one and he asked if I would like to join. I was working in Plymouth, England, trying to write a PhD thesis at night and studying for another degree on the weekends in Ireland. My Achilles was on fire at the time. I thought to myself, 'what the hell', the swimming and biking will keep me fit and I'll get by on the run with some muscle memory.

The training was miserable, especially on the bike. A painful reminder that I would have to do twice as much, at half the heart rate, to get anything close to the buzz of running. Running was heroin, triathlon was methadone, at best. The conversations got worse.

'Are you a triathlete?'

'No, I'm a runner (wish I was), I just do this when I'm injured.'

'What's a good swim time in the half-ironman?'

'I've no idea.'

'What type of bike do you have?'

'One with two wheels.'

Redemption

At this point, I had practised many different running routines. Encountered many false dawns. Slowly I began to see a colour picture, the result of many injuries and comebacks, underpinned by 3 science degrees. I began to notice how I had become adept at problem-solving long-standing injuries for international athletes and also, restoring consistent running to even the most hopeless of amateur cases. I began to wonder, could I try to love again? Re-invest once more?

Physical suffering was beginning to subside but to re-invest there would be more mental suffering to endure. As the number of injuries and the number of comebacks began to rise in tandem, a major challenge to re-investing was the reaction of friends and family. My two biggest fans are my mother and my brother, but even for them, my running had become tedious. The look in my mother's eyes was that of a woman looking at a lame dog that might be better off put down: '*Why are you doing this to yourself*?' It was almost a plead with me to stop, but stopping short in the knowledge it was a plea that would fall on deaf ears. My brother developed a reflexive roll of his eyes at my mere mention of the word running. The same gaze he uses anytime he feels something is a complete waste of time. I told friends and family less and less about it, unless I had performed well in a race. I felt better talking about it when I had concrete evidence of my progress.

I was running consistently during the Christmas of 2015. By April 2016, I was running 35:18 for 10km but more importantly, I would race 5 more times that summer – a record haul of participation. At the time I was asked what my running goals might be?

'I'd like to run a faster 10km than I did at 18 (34:40) and to be honest, if I ever broke 34, I think I'd retire.'

I returned from holidays to address part A. I committed, on the limited run training my body would tolerate, to improving every day and to having the discipline not to do too much too soon. The conversations began to change.

'Best of luck tomorrow Peter'

'Thanks.'

'Will you break 35 minutes?'

'I haven't for 12 years, but it'll give it ago.'

'Do you run?'

'Yeah.'

'What have you run?'

'I ran 34:20 for 10km *last week.'*

With Part A achieved by Christmas 2016, it was time for Part B. Consistency became the aim of the game for December and January until I moved to New Zealand for a 6-month stint in

February 2017. The challenge now was to do slightly more but be equally as consistent. I went to bed before 9pm every night and rose at 6am. Every morning, my tired old body would inevitably limp from bed. At times, the pain in my Achilles made me wonder if I was chasing an impossible dream. Warming up during an easy run used to require 1 mile, now it required 3. Initial conversations with flatmates were amusing.

'Why do you get up at 5:45am on a Saturday?'

'Because I need to be on the golf course to use the grass for barefoot running before the golfers start.'

'You've been training twice today?'

'Yes, Wednesday is double cross-trainer day, once in the morning, once in the evening.'

'Do you train every day?'

'Yes.'

'On your own?'

'Yes.'

Eventually, after what seemed like never-ending training phases, the races came – a reprieve from the boredom consistency demands. A false start in Sydney in May (dropping out halfway into a half marathon), an under-performing 34:19 in Christchurch in June, Sydney in July was the last 10km of a standard whereby PBs were possible.

It wasn't as simple as just signing up. I would have to engage in another phase of training, during a time when friends and family were visiting for a Lions tour. I would have to reorganise my mindset and cope with the guilt arising from trying to be the best you can be when family deserve your attention too. I was touring around Auckland with them, they were having a good time and I was glad to have them. Deep down I felt guilty that wherever we went, in the back of my mind was the training I would be doing the following day.

As the race approached, I was hanging on to the training process for dear life. The goal became to protect the process at all costs. I text home for a couple of sessions to freshen up my week, and asked a colleague at the university to hold a watch at the track in order to break the solitude. I set targets such as 'make this the best yoga class you've ever done'.

I flew into Sydney on Saturday night. The flight was late and the shuttle bus took longer than expected. I stayed at a hotel on top of the start line. I warmed up with the same warm-up I'd used before every session in the last few months. My brother and uncle would be out there somewhere. A warm-up provides a platform for self-doubt to creep in.

> 'What if I do it, wouldn't it be great? What if I don't do it, there's no more races left this season. Focus, stay focused on the process not the outcome, 5:24 per mile, 6:45 per 2km.'

A quick nod to my uncle and brother who I'd spotted at the start and we're off. The internal narrative begins.

'Go fast, Peter, but not too fast. This feels alright but that group of 20 are getting away, have I f**ked it up already, too slow? Mile one: 5:11. Phew, this doesn't feel too bad, glad I'm not gone through at sub 5-minute pace. Mile two: 5:36. This hurts, but don't panic, you're just levelling off from mile 1. 4km: 13:10. Good, the target was 13:30. F**k, this really hurts now, how will you get through the next 6km? Get to 6km, if you're off pace, you can jog it home, it wasn't your day, you tried, you're retiring after this season anyway, who cares about sub-34. 6km: 20:00. Damn, you're still on track, you can't give up, you've got no excuse. Get to 8km, you always finish well from there. 27:00 at 8km, exactly on target pace. Okay, push on. There is no push on. Okay, keep rhythm and cadence to 9km and you can surge from there. 9km, f**k this, I'm retiring. Okay, if you're retiring, how fast will your last ever kilometre be? Surge! I've got nothing. Okay, make the form of a sprinter and maintain cadence. Where the f**k is the clock? There it is on the left, I can see 41 seconds. I've hardly run 34:41; I couldn't have dropped off that much, could I?'

"And another one under 34", said the race announcer. A big hug for my uncle and brother, tears fill my eyes and quickly give way to a smile. Nil Desperandum indeed, 10 years on.

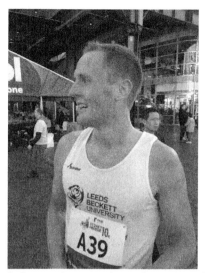

The joy and relief after running 33:46 (10-km) in Sydney after 6-months of intense training in New Zealand. Photo taken by John Francis.

12.

I remember an unfamiliar sense of pressure the night before the 2016 Abbey Dash 10km (Leeds, UK). Never before had my training preparations gone exactly as I had planned. At the same time, I wasn't quite sure what to expect because the running programme I had used to prepare looked nothing like a running programme. In fact, of the 10 sessions in a week, only 3 of them could be considered traditional running sessions. It was an experiment of sorts. What would happen if I could complete this programme for 8 weeks in a row without interruption? The answer was a first 10km personal best (34:20) in 11 years. I was no longer an injury-prone runner but instead, an athlete in training.

One of the most painful aspects of being so injury prone over such a long period of time was the gradual erosion of my identity as a runner. It becomes harder and harder to refer to yourself as a runner when you are not running very much. Ironically, this was a necessary step in becoming a consistent runner. A runner is always trying to run and be a runner. The result of this is always evaluating yourself in terms of how much and how fast you are running and how that compares to your own best and that of others (Chapter 2). This means designing training programmes which very much focus on running.

An athlete, on the other hand, looks at components of fitness rather than modes of training. An athlete asks questions such as: how can I improve these components of fitness? What needs to be done for me to move forward from where I am right now? How can I design a programme that will facilitate continual improvement whilst being adaptable to bumps in the road? If there are aspects of fitness I cannot work on right now (e.g. running) can I make gains in other areas that will help me down the line? Are there multiple ways of improving the same component of fitness? What needs to be done in order to ensure I have the lowest risk of injury possible?

In the autumn of 2016, I began to ask myself these questions. By relinquishing the possibility of ever being a competitive runner, I had inadvertently freed myself from the runner's way of thinking. When I wrote down all of the components of fitness that I felt needed to be addressed in order for me to be able to do 'some' running, there was already 4-days training on a page. This meant there was only room for 3-days of running. The result was a programme unlike anything you're likely to see in '*Runners World*'. The next page highlights the 8-week programme that facilitated a sense of uncertain expectation the night before my race in 2016.

Monday	Tuesday	Wednesday	Thursday	Friday	Saturday	Sunday	Total
Injury Prevention (40 min) • Hurdle Drills • Hip Strength • Calf Raises	Plyometric (45 min) • 2 miles • 3 x 5 Bound • 3 x 10 Ankle Hop • 5 x 60m hill sprint @ max speed	9 mile intensive aerobic or progression run. • Depending on feel working down from 7 minute/mile to 6 minute / mile.	Circuit Training (60 min) • Warm-up as per Monday. • 3 – 5 exercises. • 10 – 15 repetitions. • 3 – 4 sets.	Yoga (60 min)	-3 mile warm up & drills. -2 mile tempo effort. -5km park run at tempo pace (fastest: 17:25)	10 – 12 mile long run (easy pace).	Mileage: 32 Mileage with cross trainer: 38
Cross Trainer • 30 min	Cross Trainer • 30 min	Yoga Class (60 min)					

112

On Monday, the components of fitness addressed are mobility, endurance and recovery. The ability to move well is important for a runner, especially for the modern runner who spends large amounts of time seated. Cross training is used to mimic the running action, improve endurance and facilitate recovery without any repetitive impact. Monday generally felt like recovery, as there was nothing too physically or mentally taxing. This allowed me to top up my headspace (Chapter 8) after demanding training on the weekend and get a foothold in the working week without feeling too much training pressure that day.

Tuesday was dedicated to strength and power development using a combination of short hill repetitions, bounding and plyometric activities.[74] These activities also allowed me to use muscles in a way that would never be facilitated by ordinary running (Chapter 4). My endurance was supplemented by further work on the cross-trainer, minus the repetitive impact.

Wednesday was the first day that looks closer to something you might see in a magazine. A 9-mile intensive run was used to build endurance. Yoga is used to further mobility goals but more so to train the mind. I began to realise that yoga was the only time I was completely relaxed other than when I was asleep.[75] This ability to relax is an important component of recovery and I feel it helped to facilitate better sleep afterwards.

Thursday was a useful way of doing more intense training while remaining at a lower injury risk. Circuit training also helped me to become more conditioned and able to tolerate running. This session was used to get my muscles burning and heart rate soaring in the way that an interval session might but without the risk of injury. Interval training came later, but it was wise to become more conditioned first. There are specific adaptations in the muscle from intense circuit training that facilitate endurance performance,[76] meaning it is not simply an injury prevention exercise. It can help you run faster.

Friday used yoga for the same purpose as Wednesday and, as you can probably gather, it is essentially a recovery day – a chance to reward myself for my efforts that week and to top up headspace prior to a big weekend of training.

Saturday & Sunday: These two days form the bulk of the running programme. A classic threshold run between 3 and 5 miles at a pace slightly slower than race pace. I didn't know what this was prior to the race so I just ran at what felt like a moderate sustainable effort (~17:25) pace. Sunday was a long slow run (7-7:30-minute miles), usually barefoot and on grass. I used this to build endurance whilst having variability underfoot.[5]

Why is this concept important?
Becoming an athlete in training is important because:
(a) It facilitates consistent running more often and therefore, performance improvement.

(b) If you lose patience and want to up your training, there are ways to up training without upping injury risk.

(c) If you get injured, most of your training week is still intact, so you can continue to train as normal minus the running while you work on a solution. You can also look to develop and refine modes of training that will benefit your running long term.

(d) If you get injured; it is psychologically far less stressful which promotes acceptance and recovery much faster than if you are a runner who only runs (Chapter 9).

Application for the everyday runner to the elite

If you are someone who aims to run 30 minutes three days a week, the concept of becoming an athlete in training may seem a bit intense for your needs. I would urge you to understand the concepts rather than focus on my personal programme. For you, it may be a case of starting to run for 15 minutes on 3 days of the week and using the other 15 minutes to work on the other components of fitness. If you are an elite athlete, you are likely in a 7-day programme and it is merely a case of moving the pieces of the jigsaw around to meet your needs. If you are an elite athlete reading this book, it suggests you are an elite athlete who is injury prone in which case giving way on some of your running and replacing it with some of the ideas in this chapter might unlock the door to consistency.

Summary

- Letting go of the identity of being a 'runner' in favour of being an athlete is the first step in establishing consistent running.
- It is important to ask yourself what components of fitness need to be improved rather than how many miles you need to run.
- Weigh up the physiological gain from training against its potential physical cost i.e. interval training vs. circuit training.
- If the urge to increase training volume arises prematurely, do it via non-running-related means.
- If you pick up an injury continue to perform the non-running-related training activities as normal and seek to make performance gains while dealing with the injury.

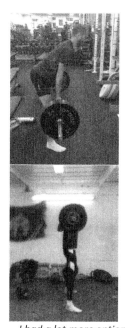
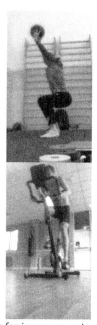

I had a lot more options for improvement as an athlete (2016-2019) compared to when I was a runner.

13.

I had never really felt my buttock muscles working before until I was walking upstairs the day after performing squat exercises for the first time. My glutes were sore, yet I felt as though my new-found muscles were powering me up the steps at the same time. Perhaps because I could feel them, I could use them. I began to notice these muscles during uphill sections on my runs too. Around the same time, I learned to sprint. The day after sprinting, the pleasant soreness in my glutes would also spread all the way down the backs of my thighs (hamstrings). And this sensation would spread all the way to my calfs when I first began to barefoot run. I don't recall the exact day when I realised squats, hill running, sprinting and barefoot running were all versions of the same thing but when I did, I had understood the concept of how to make muscles work at the same time as introducing variability to training. Variability really is a runner's best friend.

Variability underpins life itself; without genetic variation we would have died out as a species long ago. By the same token, too much genetic variation and we would no longer be identifiable as a species. Therefore, there is a sweet spot between too little and too much variation. This concept holds true for human health and disease (including running injury). To understand this concept let's use our most important muscle: the heart. We exert little conscious control over our heart but if it were to vary wildly in its rhythm, we would become acutely aware of it: i.e. there is too much variability. Conversely, people who spend a lot of time in high stress (fight or flight mode) due to poor sleep, diet, working patterns, dysfunctional relationships, isolation or a lack of physical activity have very low heart rate variability. Low heart rate variability is associated with an increased risk of depression, anxiety, cardiovascular disease and death.[77] A healthy level of heart rate variability means you can switch between stress (when required) and relaxation; meaning you do not spend too long in one state. This concept has been born out in several well-known diseases. Too little growth hormone results in dwarfism but too much can result in cancer.[78] Too high a craving for neurochemicals in the brain can lead to addiction but too little of these can lead to depression.[79] Too little inflammation impairs healing but too much creates secondary complications.[80]

Of course, we are not just biological systems running according to a genetic code, but rather biological systems interacting with our environment. Mounting evidence would suggest that too little variability in our environment can also negatively impact our health. To illustrate this concept let's use the example of diet.[81] As hunter-gatherers (most of human existence), humans ate a highly varied diet according to seasonal variation and availability.[2] As we discussed in Chapter 1, it was not until recently (~10,000 years ago) that farming was invented and began to produce a less nutritionally variable diet. Since then our diet has become increasingly processed and less nutritionally diverse. Globalisation has meant that it doesn't really vary according to season in the western world either. For example, you can eat strawberries 12 months of the year, not just in summer.

Variability and the Athlete

You can probably guess what I am going to say here. Too little stress (training) and we do not adapt (get fit) and too much stress and we are fatigued, sore and at an increased risk of injury and illness. However, an athlete rarely reaches the absolute maximum volume of training their body can tolerate. Why then, are so many fatigued, sore and injured? And why is there a need for this book? The reason is often not over-training but doing too much of the same training. It is akin to our dietary example above. Poor gut health is not always simply a case of eating too much but eating too much of the same thing. Modern humans experience little in the way of movement variability in daily life and running is a repetitive movement activity that is short on variability. This is added to by doing too much of the same kind of running. As we discussed in Chapter 4, runners tend to under-use certain muscles to moderate impacts and compound this by repetition.

Generally speaking, we need to start using our bodies more like the athlete on the right and less like the athlete on the left.

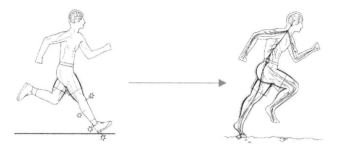

The challenge for us is to figure out diverse ways to develop the components of fitness associated with running and to integrate as many different types of running into our routine as possible. This will increase muscle work, add variability to training and allow recovery (rather than rest, chapter 5) of one system while training another. The challenge in doing this is to find our sweet spot. For example, if we were to use squats, rock climbing and yoga as our training plan we would have lots of variability in training, but we would no longer be runners.

On the next page, you will see examples of how I made better use of my muscles during running and outside of it. Can you spot what every image has in common?

(a) Double leg squats
(b) Single leg squats
(c) Dynamic bounds
    (frog jumps)
(d) Hill sprints
(e) Barefoot running
(f) Better running
    form / mechanics

Photographs taken by Tom
Bradshaw and Tim Fforde

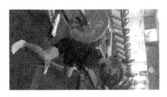

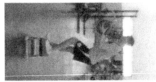

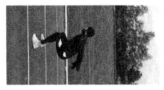

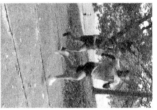

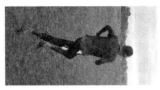

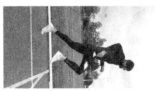

Notice how a single-leg squat, a hill run, sprinting, barefoot running and bounding-type exercises encourage bend at the hip, knee and ankle which create a spring-like action during running. This allows the muscles on the front and back of our body to work in a co-ordinated and balanced way to moderate impacts.

In Chapter 12, we used my 10km plan from 2016 to illustrate the concept of becoming an athlete in training. In this chapter, we will use one of my 10km plans from 2017 to demonstrate the concept of variability in training. You will note that the concepts from the year before are still present, but our focus in this chapter is on the origin of variability.

February – March 2017

	Monday	Tuesday	Wednesday	Thursday	Friday	Saturday	Sunday	Avg. Miles
Session 1	**Weight Training** • Squat; 80 – 95kg; 3x6 • Dead Lift, 60 – 65kg; 3 x6 • Calf Raise; 3 x12; 15kg or 3 x 1min hold (squat weight)	9 miles Rolling Hills (Golf course; barefoot)	5 miles (Golf course; barefoot)	4 – 6 miles Drills Plyometrics 2 – 6 x 400m (78 sec)	YOGA (60-minutes)	• 4-miles warm up • 4 x 7 minutes • Pace: 6:15, 6:00, 5:45, 5:35, • Road: racing flats.	10 – 12 miles (Golf course; barefoot)	35-miles
Session 2		YOGA (60-minutes)	20 – 30-minute swim		**Weight Training** (as per Monday)			

The focus on Monday is primarily strengthening the muscles I want to use during running. A by-product of Monday's session is that it also encourages development of my movement abilities due to the positions I need to get into when performing some of the exercises. As there is no running involved, it also introduces non-running variability into training.

Tuesday uses a combination of being barefoot (allowing 33 joints to move) on a variable surface (grass) and running over an undulating route to add significant within-running variability. Contrast this to a run wearing shoes, on a concrete path with little variability in undulation and it is not hard to see how the same run can be very different in terms of variability.[5] Tuesday evening develops mobility and mindfulness; a more sophisticated form of recovery than just plain old rest.

Wednesday is a short run like Tuesday followed by a swim to aid recovery. The swim introduces variability in how I'm using my body whilst also adding another small dose of endurance training.

Following an extended warm-up (building sports-specific endurance), Thursday consists of explosive exercises and the introduction of a small volume of interval running. The explosive exercises help to develop that spring-like function of the leg. It is akin to making Monday's weight sessions more dynamic, closer towards the movement intended – a moving strength session. The speed required by interval repetitions again encourages a more spring-like use of the lower leg but also adds variability in terms of the running form and speed required. The explosive nature of Thursday's training also builds confidence in my body's capabilities (discussed in Chapter 14). The small dose of interval training is respecting the slow and steady build-up required for consistent running (discussed more in Chapter 15).

Why is this concept important?

Variability in training is important because:

(e) It reduces overload to any one area of your musculoskeletal system.

(f) It facilitates recovery without the risks associated with complete rest.

(g) It is mentally stimulating. This helps to reduce boredom in training.

(h) It negates the repetitive nature of running and encourages the use of muscles in different ways.

(i) If you live in the western world, the use of transport, chairs and other sustained postures means there is likely little variability in your day.

(j) It contributes to becoming an athlete in training (Chapter 11).

Application for the everyday runner to the elite

If you are someone who aims to run 30 minutes on 3 days of the week, the concept of variability in training may seem like a lot more work than you have time for. As we discussed in the last chapter, you may introduce this concept via splitting your

30-minute session in two. But there are opportunities for variability throughout the entirety of your day. Parking further away from work and walking adds variability due to the different biomechanics used in walking. Getting a standing desk at work allows you alternate between sitting and standing during the day which adds variability and some conditioning to your lower limbs. Running for 15 x 1minute fast, 1minute slow instead of 30-minutes straight adds variety to running and often reduces the soreness associated with repetition.

If you are an elite athlete or a competitive amateur, like I was, it is best to introduce the concept into your lifestyle according to the facilities you have available. You can also ask a coach to come up with some within-running variety in sessions and ordinary runs.

Summary

- Variability is key to human health. Too much or too little variability in our physiological systems can lead to acute or chronic disease.

- Low environmental variability (diet, exercise, sitting) can overload certain systems.

- Runners tend to do too much of the same training.

- Different training (strength, yoga, cross-training) and different types of running (sprinting, hill running, barefoot running) can be used to increase variability in a runner's plan.

- Adding variability to everyday life is especially important for those living a western lifestyle

14.

Sprinting up that hill as fast as I could, I knew it wasn't possible for there to be anything 'wrong' with my legs. Yes, my tendon was a bit sore, but it was clearly working extremely well. This was further confirmed by my ability to hop and bound; to perform calf raises with 100-kg on my shoulders and to do track sessions for the first time in 6-years. I was beginning to develop (or redevelop) a confidence in my body's capabilities. When other small niggles would develop, I didn't panic. I modified training for a day or two but ultimately, I knew my body was more than capable of what I was doing. I started to see consistency in training as a given. I knew this was the case when I started to think more about what races I would do and when, rather than whether my body would hold up or not. I had established a 'new normal'.

The amount of time a runner misses out on training is more closely associated with what they think about pain and how that makes them behave than the structural 'damage' offered by diagnosis (Chapter 7). According to evidence,[67] the improvements in my athletic capabilities above were as much due to the following as any physical changes;

- A reduction in psychological distress when experiencing pain

- A subsequent reduction in avoiding activities due to fear-based beliefs

- An increased confidence in my ability to manage pain

- More positive coping strategies

The meaning we attribute to an event, in this case pain associated with running, influences the amount of psychological distress we experience. Psychological distress can amplify our experience of pain. The amount of psychological distress we experience determines how likely we are to avoid or develop fear in relation to certain activities. The amount of time we spend avoiding activities determines the amount of 'rest' (Chapter 5) our musculoskeletal system receives and how deconditioned we become. In a nutshell, this was the message of Chapter 7. Undoing this cycle and arriving at the positive changes described above can prove difficult but let's have a look at the elements that led to me experiencing less distress, less avoidance, more confidence and a greater ability to navigate setbacks. To do this, I contrasted my experience of pain during the years I was injured (2004-2016) and during the years I was consistent (2016-2019).

The changes described in the table on the next page, appear to be quite straightforward, and they are, but let's look at the elements of my training programme that make these changes easier. To illustrate this, we will use the training week from Chapter 12.

Pain	Meaning	Threat	Distress	Pain	Behaviour
2004 - 2016	Certain injury (diagnosis and abnormality, Ch. 3) Time off running Loss of identity Loss of control over physical and mental health Loss of social status Loss of performance goals Loss of training targets Experience of shame	Extremely high	Profound	Increases	Deny the experience. Make pain worse Pursue complex / expensive treatment Increased junk food consumption Increased alcohol consumption Decreased physical activity
2016 - 2019	A change in perception of discomfort that day Modified running or cross training Identity maintained Control of physical and mental health maintained Performance goals still intact Training targets modified No shame	Low	Low	Stays the same or lowers	Modify running and/or introduce added cross training Maintain normal non-running components of training Add a new component to training due to increased time Maintain normal dietary and physical activity habits Use the opportunity to improve other aspects of performance

Monday	Tuesday	Wednesday	Thursday	Friday	Saturday	Sunday	Total
Injury Prevention (40 min) • Hurdle Drills • Hip Strength • Calf Raises	Plyometric (45 min) • 2 miles • 3 x 5 Bound • 3 x 10 Ankle Hop • 5 x 60m hill sprint @ max speed	9 mile intensive aerobic or progression run. • Depending on feel working down from 7 minute/mile to 6 minute / mile.	Circuit Training (60 min) • Warm-up as per Monday. • 3 – 5 exercises. • 10 – 15 repetitions. • 3 – 4 sets.	Yoga (60 min)	-3 mile warm up & drills. -2 mile tempo effort. -5km park run at tempo pace (fastest: 17:25)	10 – 12 mile long run (easy pace).	Mileage: 32 Mileage with cross trainer: 38
Cross Trainer • 30 min	Cross Trainer • 30 min	Yoga Class (60 min)					

Imagine during this week I experience pain associated with slow or steady running (the most common type of running-associated pain). Monday is not affected, Tuesday is not affected, Wednesday morning needs to be modified, Wednesday evening is not affected, Thursday is not affected, Friday is not affected, Saturday and Sunday need to be modified. Straight away my level of psychological distress will be less because my entire training week is not dependent solely on slow or steady running. Between 2004-2016, I was losing close to 100% of my training week whereas between 2016-2019 I am only losing or modifying 30% of my weekly training load. Psychological distress will be hugely influenced by the size of the loss. Thanks to understanding the benefits of being an athlete in training (Chapter 11) and the importance of variability (Chapter 12) in training I can never lose out in the way I used to; this immediately makes things easier.

Another way to lower psychological distress when experiencing pain is to have activities, outside of typical running sessions, which allow you to demonstrate your physical capabilities. This provides reassurance that your body, generally speaking, is working well and niggles will subside. Let's use Tuesday as an example. Imagine I experience pain (previously meaning injury) but I am still able to sprint, hop and bound or lift a heavy weight. It is difficult to feel injured when such maximal effort activities are still possible. This helps you to see your experience of pain or the niggle as a part of you that can be managed rather than a signifier of your injury status.

To summarise this section, the level of threat is lower because the size of the loss and the level of uncertainty are reduced by three things:

(a) The training programme is not solely dependent on running.

(b) The training programme includes elements that allow the runner to demonstrate physical competence in the presence of pain.

(c) Fewer complex diagnosis and interventions have been pursued.

Combined this leads to less psychological distress and therefore, lower pain sensitivity.

Why is this concept important?

Establishing a new normal is important because:

(a) It reduces the loss experienced by the runner during pain or injury.

(b) It provides the runner with alternatives outside of running.

(c) It allows the runner to demonstrate competence in the use of their body despite interruption due to pain or injury.

(d) It reduces psychological distress and therefore pain sensitivity which reduces time spent on negative coping strategies.

Application for the everyday runner to the elite

If you are someone who aims to run 30 minutes on 3 days of the week, but due to the learnings in this book have decided to split that session into 15 minutes of non-running and running-related activities you will simply be able to increase the duration of non-running-related activities. This will give you a focus while you seek advice on the management of your pain or injury. If you are a competitive amateur or elite athlete, you can get creative in relation to the different forms of training you can use to modify existing training and demonstrate physical competence. Activities I have not mentioned include swimming, cycling, walking and rock climbing. There is no right or wrong answer provided you understand the concept you are trying to introduce and why you are introducing it.

Summary

- The meaning we attribute to pain significantly alters the level of threat detected by our brain and the resulting psychological distress. Psychological distress can elevate pain sensitivity and lead to negative coping strategies.

- Reappraising the experience of pain as something to be managed rather than an end point (i.e. injury) can significantly limit the time lost to due to pain or injury.

- A varied training programme lowers the loss experienced due to running pain or injury.

- Training sessions which develop physical competence can boost a runner's confidence in their physical capabilities and lower the level of threat associated with pain.

15.

In chapter 12 I tell the story of my first personal best in a very long time following 8 weeks of a very unconventional run programme. The average running volume for those 8 weeks was 32 miles and in later years it reached 40 miles in similar programmes. I calculated the average weekly mileage for the 156 weeks of training I had done between 2016-2019 and it was 30 miles. The run volume was modest and the increases over time negligible, but my consistency of training was impeccable. During this period my 10km times progressed from 36:40 to 35:18 to 34:20 and to 33:46. Slow and steady had won the race. Consistency was king.

The ability to delay gratification is central to the achievement of anything worthwhile in life. Tolerating the boredom of consistently doing basics things well is central to raring our children, financial security, producing meaningful work, developing relationships with others, leading a healthy lifestyle and of course injury-free running. The good news is, you can learn to love it or, to paraphrase Victor Frankl (author of man's search for meaning)[82], learn to take pride in the suffering and the meaning it holds for you as an individual.

Developing a consistent approach to training can be seen as taming your inner chimp.[83] The chimp wants to feel good immediately and to do so it is willing to up your running volume too quickly. The chimp will even create stories to make you think you haven't changed your loading too quickly when in reality you have. To avoid the chimp hijacking your long-term running progress there are 5 key tricks:

(a) Record the training data so that it is measurable against what you agreed with yourself before the chimp took over.

(b) Develop a set of habits so that you cannot help but do the right thing.

(c) Substitute increases in running with other forms of training when the urge to run more is strong.

(d) Distract yourself from the boredom of consistent training by finding ways to add variety.

(e) Meaning. Be clear on your why.

Write it down and do the time

For any goal you really want to achieve, you need to know the cost: write it down and do the time. In my field of sport and health science, it is not uncommon to prescribe training programmes of 6, 12 and 24 weeks. There are various physiological reasons for this including the minimum amount of time needed to see a meaningful improvement in fitness. In my experience as a runner, (the 2nd time around) I generally found 8 weeks to be a good training block in terms of letting myself get to grips with the training programme (the initial soreness, tiredness), getting to master the training programme (running well and finding things easy) and getting to have an easy week prior to a race. By the time I got to week 7/8, I was starting to find training easy and starting to get bored, but at that point I didn't have long to go, so I stuck to task. The key is to agree what the 8 weeks will look like in advance and not to deviate when the chimp gets bored. If you are frequently injured, I suggest revising your 8-week programme to the bare minimum of running. This may help you to demonstrate to yourself that you are at least capable of an 8-week uninterrupted training programme. This will build confidence in your ability to keep promises to yourself and show you that you are capable of consistency. Some runners may wonder why I do not refer to periodisation (the process of cycling training between hard and easy weeks). I find the human body does not respond to a calendar, rather to training and life-related stress. Therefore, I prefer a programme that aims for a constant moderate effort without sudden change. A flexible mindset in training means the runner can adapt training on any given week when tiredness occurs and not when the programme says they should. The power of a consistent moderate effort is highlighted below. The average mileage is around 30 as evidenced by the almost straight line anchored at the number 30 (on the left). By contrast my 10-km times are illustrated by the line that falls sharply with my increasing consistency.

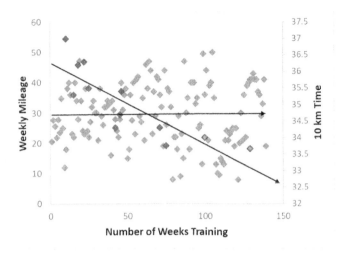

Form habits and work out the trade-offs

Morning ***cues*** you to clean your teeth (***behaviour***) to have fresh breath (*receive a **reward***). Sitting in your car *cues* the use of clutch, accelerator, and brake (*behaviour*) to get to work (*receive a reward*). If I asked you how exactly you used your tooth brush this morning and in what way you pressed the clutch or first used the brake this morning, the chances are you would not remember. You would probably offer me a generic description of what you think you normally do. This is because habits, when repeated often enough, become automatic, requiring little conscious control. This is important because when you are tired, distracted and have a million other things

140

to do (i.e. low headspace; chapter 8) you still manage to clean your teeth. Habits have made teeth cleaning automatic rather than optional. Runners need to develop habits which result in a lower risk of injury.

To illustrate the concept of writing a programme down and positive habit formation we will use my training plan from when I was attempting to run under 33minutes. This is the last training plan I followed prior to retiring from competitive running. This phase of training was 9 weeks long. It contains many of the components from Chapter 12, 13 and 14. Due to my overall level of consistency by this point (~140 weeks), I could attain this training load within 3 weeks. Once I was capable of what is written on the next page, I did not increase it for the remainder of the programme.

Monday	Tuesday	Wednesday	Thursday	Friday	Saturday	Sunday
Weights Session	Plyometrics/Bounds +	2-hour Bike ride	8-miles	Weights Session	Plyometrics/Bounds +	15-miles
O.head Squat W.Up: 1 x 12 (5kg)	Track Session	(easy recovery)	barefoot grass run	as per Monday	Tempo work & hills	
Single leg squats: 3 x 12 (6kg)	(8-km)					
Squats: 3 x 6 (95 kg)					Example:	
Deadlift from Hang: 3 x 6 (70 kg)	Example:					
Double leg calf raise: 3 x 6 (105kg)					5-km tempo effort	
	5 x 1km (3:20), 400 (75)				8 x 40 sec hill	
					3-km in 10:10	
	AM: 20 minutes app guided yoga and 3 x 12 eccentric achilles loading					
Total			40-miles and 6-hours cross training.			

You might notice that my double session days from other programmes are gone. If you study closely you will also see there are no 60-minute yoga classes or circuit training sessions. All programmes are a series of trade-offs. You cannot have everything. I frequently weighed up fitness gains against the risk of injury when deciding what my final **sustainable** programme would be. Consistency was my number one priority. In this programme, I decided to push for further improvement via the addition of a 2-hour bike ride and consistently delivering short but heavy resistance training sessions on Monday and Friday. To negate any potential downside to losing my yoga class and to ensure continuity of my Achilles tendon health, I created a new morning habit. Every morning, after my coffee I completed 20 minutes of yoga and my Achilles tendon injury-prevention routine. In this way, I had more time to pursue gains elsewhere, but I could also maintain some of the improvements I had made from previous programmes.

Distract, Distract, Distract

"Distract. Distract. Distract." This is what my grandmother used to say to my mother in relation to my brother and I. We were likely tormented toddlers and tormenting all around us.

We use distraction to negate an unpleasant experience. Watch a child who bangs its hand. The child's parent instinctively either blows on it or rubs it furiously. This form of distraction is useful because it stimulates other nerve fibres and helps to lower the intensity of the pain. However, the unpleasant experience my grandmother was attempting to distract us from was more likely boredom or fatigue. Boredom and fatigue are unpleasant experiences which accompany us most of our adult lives. They are both components of an injury-free running programme that need to be managed.

To illustrate how I have used distraction to ensure consistency in training, I will use this short story.

In July 2018, I ran a 5km race in York. It was my first race in 2018 due to undertaking an Achilles tendon rehabilitation programme (5weeks with no running) between March and May. In the race, I equalled my 5km personal best (16:10). This was surprising given the little volume of running I had completed beforehand. I ran 3 days per week. This included building a track session from 2x400m up to 12x400m (slow and steady), a 5-mile midweek run to 8 miles and an 8-mile Sunday run to 12 miles. Without a single continuous tempo run or practice effort, I was running as fast as I ever had.

How? A consistency that was maintained and enhanced by distraction. I powered through the period from March to May of that year using a cross-training programme and an athlete in training mindset (Chapter 11). This works well for short periods (1-8 weeks) but becomes difficult to maintain for longer periods. By May I was still fit as a result of my initial efforts, but I was getting bored and in need of another distraction. I signed up to a half-Ironman triathlon with my cousin which was due to take place on July 29th. As a result, when I ran 16:10 for 5km in York, I could also swim 2km and cycle 80km comfortably. The beauty of the triathlon distraction was that it allowed me to build my running at a pace my legs were happy with. In other words, the development of a consistent running routine was disguised amongst a triathlon routine. The swimming and biking helped me stay fit and mentally feel like I was working hard. As the weeks went by, my running was beginning to build. (Note: *learning new skills besides running is important for runners in need of distraction*).

March to July was a series of distractions that helped me to bridge the gap from no running towards consistent running again. There was no pause in my training and so my 5km performance was most likely a product of my efforts over the last 3 years: a consistent, moderate, and sometimes unpleasant effort.

Find your WHY

The only thing that can hold a long-term goal together is meaning. In my case, there was huge meaning derived from attaining consistent running when I could not for the previous 12 years. This was added to by a desire to break my 10km personal best from when I was an 18-year-old and subsequently to run under 34 minutes for the distance. Although I was grateful to achieve my performance targets, the major success of this story was running for all but 8 of 156 weeks and to retire on my own terms. You might have a similar goal to overcome injury, to feel better, to perform better or to be a better person through engaging in a fitness activity you enjoy. Whatever it is, you need to find it. Dare I say, if you don't like running, you'll struggle to overcome injury. To achieve consistency will require good habits and a slow and steady approach. There will be lots of boredom and fatigue to manage, so make sure you know why you're doing it.

Why is this concept important?

To be able to sustain an effort for long periods of time is important because:

(a) All meaningful goals are achieved via consistently doing basic things well.

(b) An inability to delay gratification will lead to injury.

(c) It promotes habit formation, we are what we repeatedly do, excellence is a habit and therefore, so is injury-free running.

Application for the everyday runner to the elite

If you are someone who aims to run 30 minutes on 3 days of the week, take your time building up to that level. Write down (or have someone help you) a gradually progressive programme over the course of 6-8 weeks and stick to it. Develop good habits around your running such as the inclusion of pre- and post-run mobility. Prepare for the fact that when you reach your goal, you will become bored. Rather than increasing the volume of running (which you can also do carefully) try changing one of your 30-minute runs into a hill session or an interval session. This will help distract you into consistently completing your 30 minutes on 3 days per week while increasing overall fitness. If you are a competitive amateur or elite athlete, the same rules apply. Write down the minimum training you are confident you can complete and stick to it for 8 weeks. Refine your habits and distract yourself into ever-increasing consistency. Be clear on your why.

Summary

- Our inner chimp desires instant gratification (sudden increases in training volume).

- Writing a plan when you have clarity of thought will give you something to refer to when the chimp attempts to hijack your efforts.

- Habits can make positive behaviours automatic and help to increase headspace.

- Consistency can lead to boredom and commitment fatigue. It can be useful to have other goals and forms of training to distract us.

- It is important for our running to have clear meaning for us to stick to task.

- Runners should note how fast they can run from so little training when it is done consistently and supplemented with distraction.

Sept 10th   Project sub·33   Oct 1st   2018

Mon   Weights   Mon: Weights
Tue   Track   Tue   Track
Wed   Easy   Wed: Yoga Bike
Thur Weights   Thur Alt - 8
Fri   Tempo   Fri   Weights 1 Hour Circuit
Sat   Long Run   Sat   Tempo
Sun   Rest   Sun: Long Run

Sept 17th   Oct 8th (Dublin Weekend).

Mon: Weights   Mon   Weights
Tue   Track   Tue: Track
Wed: Easy   Wed: Yoga · Easy 8 Bike.
Thur: Weights   Thur Weights Easy 8
Fri. Bike   Fri   Tempo Weights
Sat   Tempo   Sat   Long. Tempo
Sun. Long Run   Sun   Rest   Long Run

Sept 24th   Oct 15th

Mon   Weights (Phil won)   Mon: Weights
Tue   Track   Tue   Track.
Wed   Yoga   Wed   Yoga · Bike
Thur Alt - 8   Thur Alt 8
Fri, Weights 1 Hour Circuit Fri Weights 1 Hour Circuit
Sat   Tempo   Sat: Tempo
Sun   Long Run   Sun   Long Run

Oct 22nd   Mon Rest   Thur Alt - 10k
(Alt Week).   Tue Track   Fri   Weights
                  Wed Yoga Bike   Sat   Tempo
                                     Sun   Medium Run

Into my 3rd of year of consistency in 2018. I could literally write it down and do the time. Interestingly, injury or being able to train was never a concern by this point. It was all about how fast I would run.

148

16.

I was once asked at a talk what was the first thing I did when I was aiming to run well. Without thinking I answered, 'finish work by 4pm'. I think the audience member was expecting an answer that involved a specific training routine, but the answer I gave was a serious one. Without enough 'headspace' consistent running is very difficult to achieve. I would finish at 4 because I knew that gave me enough time to prepare a good meal, anticipate any logistical issues for training in the coming days, relax and in turn, get a good night's sleep. Finishing work on time or early was key to effective planning, nutrition, relaxation and sleep – a potent combination for injury prevention and general well-being.

My English teacher warned us before our exams about the dangers of 'knowing a little bit of everything and not a lot about anything'. To live in 2021 is to be trying to do a bit of everything and ending up with not very much of anything. Always in a rush, we are increasingly disconnected from ourselves and those around us. To simplify, we increasingly live in our heads and focus on what we perceive we must do at the expense of how our bodies feel. Findings ways to slow down and increase headspace is therefore the first step in becoming an injury free runner.

Limit Your Options

There are only a certain number of things we can do well. Accepting this was one of the first things that put me on the road to consistency. I had the capacity to perform at work and do my training well. I was a pitch-side therapist for my local rugby club on a Saturday. This also served as a weekly social event and a chance to have a couple of beers and relax. These activities represented a typical week during training blocks. There was little room for anything else. There were sacrifices to be made, with trips to follow my favourite football and rugby teams needing to be put on hold. It wasn't so much the games themselves, but the headspace involved in going there and back and the disruption to routine that would spill over into the following week. If running is an important activity to you, give it the time it deserves, not just the minutes you are running. Limit your options.

ABC: Anticipation Breeds Consistency

If I had an ABC acronym, it would be the above. Consistency on a given day or week starts the night or week before. We need to learn to anticipate bottle necks in work, block out diary time or change training days in advance of problems occurring. For example, when travelling with work, you could check your schedule and the hotel facilities in order to determine when you will train. This would be instead of passively showing up and returning home with a list of excuses as to why your training was not complete.

This concept might apply to you getting a moderate dose of running done more regularly and consistently (hence lowering injury risk) or to getting those rehabilitation exercises or yoga sessions done that you can never find the time to. Anticipation is central to achieving consistent injury-free running.

What you must do versus what you think you must do

In work or life, can you tell the difference between what you have to do and what you perceive you have to do? In my experience, for most people, there is always a mismatch between these two things. Generally, people overestimate what they must do. The reality of what they must do is much smaller. To use one definition of anxiety, it is 'an overestimation of what is going to happen and underestimation of the ability to cope'. We live in anxious times.

In most cases, with some exceptions, if people no longer stayed late at work – the world would keep turning, but it is often difficult for people to see this. Granted, if you conduct open heart surgery, I suggest you close the patient's chest before going home or if you have kids waiting for you at the school gates, I suggest you collect them, but after examples such as these it starts to get very grey in relation to what 'must be done' (other than die).

Knowing the difference between these two things is fundamental to limiting options, blocking out diary time and anticipating bottle necks. These must all be negotiated to ensure consistent running.

Why is this concept important?

Finding ways to increase headspace is important because:

(a) It increases the ability to delay gratification.
(b) It reduces stress and therefore inflammation and chronic pain.
(c) It allows you to anticipate barriers to consistency and plan for them.
(d) It allows you to more clearly differentiate between what you must do and what you think you must do.

Application for the everyday runner to the elite

If you are someone who aims to run 30 minutes on 3 days of the week, this chapter was written for you. You might find that some weeks you run 3 days and other weeks you run none. The fluctuations in training load using this approach heightens the possibility of pain, soreness, stiffness, along with injury and the negative psychological consequences associated. This chapter teaches you the concepts to get your running and what needs to be done around it on a more even keel. If you are a competitive amateur or elite athlete, the chances are you also need to juggle competing demands. Use this chapter to interpret the concepts and apply them to prioritise your busy training schedule.

Summary

- Modern life moves at a speed which headspace for meaningful activities.
- A conscious decision to limit the number of opt. our daily lives is essential to enjoyable and injury-running.
- Building discipline over time by starting small is important for runners with competing demands in their lives.
- Anticipation breeds consistency. It is important to anticipate bottle necks and adapt the training routine accordingly.
- It is important to learn the difference between what you must do and what you perceive you must do in order to create more headspace.

17.

I was in pain and living in a desert with no access to physical therapies. I knew what was wrong. It was plantar fasciitis, the familiar heel pain that had taken months of rest and shockwave therapy to resolve previously. I was teaching English in Qatar, the year after my first degree and running was my release. I didn't hold out much hope of a resolution. A friend back in Ireland sent me a magazine article about the benefits of barefoot running. I had nothing to lose. I drove to the only grass park in the country, took off my shoes and ran for 15 minutes. The second time I did this, my pain had vanished. At the time, to me, it was a medical miracle. On return to Ireland to start my PhD, I enthusiastically told my professor what had happened on my middle-eastern adventure. He was sceptical but he agreed to allow one of his final-year undergraduate students to investigate the topic as part of their research project. In short, we found that runners ran differently when barefoot, especially at slow speeds. This study has since been published. Later, I encountered more runners who experienced the immediate resolution of plantar fasciitis from barefoot running, I published their data as medical case reports. Recently, I observed adolescents in New Zealand happily run distances of up to 3,000m barefoot on a hard tartan track. I also published this observation. During my consistent streak, I ran up to 20 miles at sub-3-hour marathon pace barefoot. It is fair to say that being barefoot played a significant role in the resolution of my running injuries.

Have you ever breathed a sigh of relief when you've come home after a long day and kicked off your shoes? Have you ever noticed when you are barefoot on the grass of a park or the sand of a beach, it inherently feels good? Have you ever observed a toddler scream because they don't want to put their shoes on?

If the answer to any of those questions is yes, you inherently understand your evolutionary legacy. You don't need a scientist to tell you what inherently feels good. The nerve receptors in your feet are the same type that are found in your hands. Imagine if I was trying to use my fingers with the same dexterity, as I am when typing these words, but I had a pair of sandals attached to my hands. This is what it is like for the foot that lives in shoes.

I have written extensively in this book about an increasing disconnection from our bodies and how that manifests in mental and physical illness. The feet are our only connection with the ground below us. Yoga and mindfulness practitioners know that in order to feel grounded, you must remove your shoes. It is also a pre-requisite for better balance.[84]

The Mind-Body Connection

Why do we feel and move better when barefoot? The human foot comprises of 26 bones and 33 joints. This fact alone tells us it is a complex structure capable of many, many variations of subtle movements. The skin that covers these bones deforms in response to pressure and reforms when the pressure is released. This property is present in every human tissue (e.g. heart, lungs and muscle). The nerves underneath our skin are stimulated according to the amount of pressure, stretch and tension experienced by the skin. These nerves send a rich source of information to our spinal cord and brain. Our spinal cord and brain can then signal to a variety of muscles to make small or large refinements depending on the stimulation coming from the ground.[5] Therefore, balance tends to be better barefoot.[84] A bit like a computer, the higher the quality of input, the better the output. The next time you walk barefoot on an uneven surface (sand is a good example) watch how the feet and toes change and deform slightly differently with every step. This means that the communication to the brain is slightly different with each step and the movement strategy slightly more refined. You may remember from chapter 12 that variability is key to health, and to be barefoot is to experience variability. In shoes, walking on concrete, the complex anatomy of our foot becomes redundant and the quality of information to the brain quite blunt. The resulting movement strategies also become quite blunt. You may have heard of the phrase, use it or lose it, in relation to muscles and exercise. This is certainly

156

true of the muscles in our feet. Wearing shoes causes the muscles in our feet to become smaller and weaker as they are not being used.[57] Adults who transition from traditional footwear to minimalist footwear see increases in foot muscle size and strength in just 8 weeks from having to use their foot again.[85] Similarly, older adults demonstrate improvements in balance in minimalist footwear potentially reducing falls risk.[86] Children who take part in a school-based barefoot running programme demonstrate better sprint biomechanics and jump height performance compared to a control group wearing shoes.[87] Anecdotally, children in shoeless classrooms demonstrate better behaviour and parents of children with some forms of autism are reporting better behaviour in their children when not wearing traditional footwear (our research group is currently designing experiments in this area).

Should I run barefoot?

Unlike your hunter-gatherer ancestors or the adolescents I recently studied in New Zealand, you most likely have not grown up barefoot or with minimalist foot coverings. If you have reached adulthood and live in an industrialised country, it is highly likely that both your everyday shoes and sport shoes contain some form of heel that has held your calf and Achilles tendon complex in a shortened position for most of your life. The sole of your shoe and the associated arch support means you most likely have weakened foot muscles also. If you have spent a lot of time in fashionable shoes, there is a good chance that the shape of your foot is nothing like those seen in habitually barefoot populations. The result of all this bad news is that if you were to immediately run barefoot, your foot would experience a loading like nothing it has experienced since you were a toddler (remember the lesson of Chapter 1). Just like training, the process of being barefoot requires a slow and steady approach and is influenced by many factors.

In my case, I was 23 when I discovered barefoot running and, to be honest, I found the transition into running barefoot very straight-forward. I had youth on my side and my tall frame (195cm, 6ft. 4in) seemed to appreciate the shorter stride and pliable grass surface I was running on. I had some initial discomfort, post-running, in my calves but that was about it. Even the discomfort I experienced was positive, like after having a strong massage or doing a good workout. It was in stark contrast to the soreness and stiffness I had in my calves from logging miles in standard running shoes. I found this experience to be replicated in runners I worked with who also suffered with plantar fasciitis. It seems that runners with this condition are prone to over-stride and land heavily on the heel, two things cushioned shoes encourage.

Not everyone will have the experience that I and my fellow heel pain sufferers had, especially if someone is older. With aging, the speed of recovery from strenuous exercise of any kind is reduced. In addition, older adults will have been wearing traditional footwear for a longer period of time prior to their transition to minimalist activities. Combined, this means they are more prone to injury from sudden changes in workload.

I would encourage people to spend as much time as possible barefoot but not necessarily running or walking long distances to begin with. Be barefoot around the house and in the back garden. Start to wear minimalist footwear in the office. Start to add in some barefoot walking on the beach or in the park. Build your minutes the same way this book advises you to build your training load.

If I don't run barefoot, what should I run in?

I did my road or track-based training sessions and ran my fastest ever race (2017) in a pair of shoes that were light, comfortable and cost me £27. I ran the following season in a similar pair that cost me £32. At public talks, I explain my 3 criteria as light (I can feel what's happening), comfortable (it makes inherent sense) and cheap (the price of a shoe makes no difference). You could say my 3 criteria are as evidence-based as any other criteria for prescribing a specific shoe type to an individual i.e. not very evidence-based.

If you have a pair of shoes that are comfortable and are not causing you a problem, the chances are you are on to a winner. Watch out for the myth that each shoe only has a certain number of miles in them before they need to be changed. I have had a number of runners report to me clinically with an injury that results from replacing their worn-out shoes (changing the load to the foot too quickly). Again, I ran my best time with a hole in the top of both shoes. There is no limit to the number of miles a shoe can do other than when it falls apart.

Why is this concept important?

Being barefoot is important because:

(a) Our feet are our only point of contact with the ground.

(b) The quality of information our brain and spinal cord receives is enhanced.

(c) Our foot muscles get stronger.

(d) For many runners, it causes them to adopt better running form.

Application for the everyday runner to the elite

If you are someone who aims to run 30 minutes on 3 days of the week, you almost certainly need some time to transition to barefoot activities. Start with spending more time barefoot where possible or in minimalist shoes where being barefoot is not possible. Begin walking on grass or sand-based surfaces and build your minutes slowly. Perhaps start with 15 minutes barefoot walking at the end of a longer walk. Save money on expensive running shoes by trying to find shoes that are light, comfortable and cheap. If you are a competitive amateur or elite athlete, your transition to barefoot activities will depend on a few things. How conditioned you are will be a big factor. For example, if you already perform strength and conditioning training and/or practice yoga barefoot, it may be possible to introduce a small amount of barefoot running immediately. Perhaps try to integrate barefoot running into warm-ups and cool downs. I recommend using a medium-firm grass or sand surface in this process. The pliable nature of these surfaces will allow you to run as normal without hesitation that may be present on concrete. At the same time, these surfaces are not so soft that it is like a resistance training session as would be the case with running through mud or sand dunes. If you are an elite athlete you likely have a shoe contract which means you don't waste money on shoes, so just make sure the model you use is comfortable. If you are a competitive amateur, save money using the 3 criteria.

Summary

- Humans have an inherent sense of what feels good: pay attention to it.

- The quality of information we get through the soles of our feet determines the quality of movement strategy we use subsequently.

- Children should be allowed to develop as barefoot and minimalist as possible.

- Adults require a careful transition to barefoot activities.

- Runners should aim to have shoes that are light, comfortable and cheap.

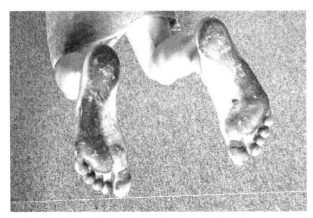

A window to the soul: *The soles of my feet tell their own story after a barefoot run in Leeds in 2018.*

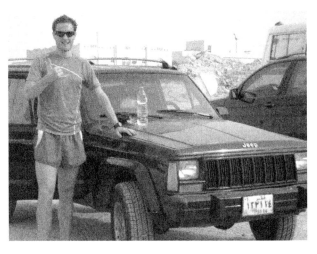

Running through the desert: *I first realised the benefits of kicking off my shoes when working in Qatar in 2010.*

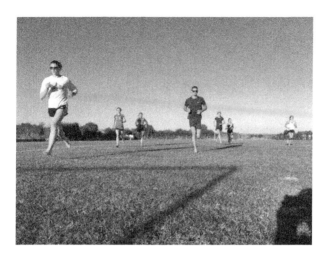

Faro, Portugal 2018: 8-years after my first barefoot run, using barefoot activities with international athletes as part of an injury prevention workshop.

18.

I still do it now: set myself a target (albeit a less ambitious one) for my running; wear a watch so that I am fed a constant stream of information about pace, distance, and heart rate; compare that to where I was, where I am and where I'm aiming for; I notice what other runners are doing on social media; I read an article that makes me feel like I should be doing something different; I am told something by someone else about how I look or how I run and take it as fact. Before I know it, my running is taking place entirely in my head. If I was asked how tired my legs were, how my pain sensitivity was, how much I was enjoying the experience of running, or how I felt running generally – I probably wouldn't be able to answer these questions. Yet, the answers to these questions are always the ones I need to modify and improve my running situation. More often than not, I need to get out of my head, ask myself how I am feeling right now and act accordingly. This has become increasingly difficult in the age of information overload.

We have already discussed in this book that the key to success is developing a set of habits that facilitate you to consistently do basic things well. After that it is all about time and patience.

As the sport scientist among my friends and family, I am frequently asked about the latest footwear, watches, nutrition, and training plans. To their surprise, my answers are usually quite simple. Here is a selection of the most common:

- Your body can adapt to perform amazing feats with training; you do not need all the gear, but you do need more training.

- 99% of your bike time in your next triathlon will be explained by the training you have done and not the cost of your bike or the type of energy gel you are using.

- If the new shoes hurt, wear the old ones.

- You can train to be able to exercise for several hours without breakfast.

- Pace and heart rate aside, how did you feel during the run?

- You might not need an MRI scan just yet.

- If your body won't be ready for that event, maybe let it go and choose another one.

The list of similar responses is endless. Seven of the 10 problem chapters in section 1 arise from being in our heads and using overly simplistic reasoning at the expense of listening to our bodies.

Summary of Section 2: How to stop running injury

The best way to reduce your risk of running injury is to have a think about the volume of training you can do right now, comfortably, no matter how small. Aim to stay with that volume for the next 4 – 8 weeks. To increase your chances of doing so, I suggest you keep a record of your training every week. Make sure you block out time for your running, so that you do not become psychologically overloaded.

Introduce variability into your training by ensuring no two days are the same e.g. avoid running the same loop or the same speed all the time. Linked to this, try adding some non-running variability into your training. This is sometimes referred to as strength and conditioning training but in reality, yoga, pilates, cross-training at the gym, circuits, weight-lifting, hill runs and sprinting are all ways of using your body differently and at higher intensities than plain old jogging. This will help you use all of your muscles more fully and reduce the risk of joints and other tissues from being overloaded.

If you live near a nice grass park or a beach with medium firm sand, try to incorporate 10 to 15-minutes of easy barefoot running as part of your warmup or cool down a couple of times per week. At least once per week, run up a hill as fast as you can (like a child on a school sports day), this will help you to increase confidence in your body and be more psychological resilient to minor injuries that occur. Be aware of other sedentary behaviours associated with our modern lives that reduce movement variability and try to interrupt them. For example, park the car a little further away from work and walk to it (walking is movement variability) or alternate between standing and seated desks.

Good luck and take your time.

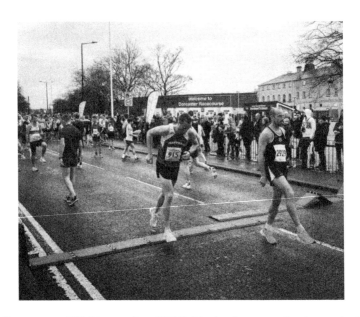

Doncaster UK, November 2018: Limbering up prior to my last race before retirement from competitive running.

This memory is bittersweet. I had trained my body to be easily capable of ≤32:50 for 10-km but my mind had had enough. Despite 14-months of high-quality training since my previous best (33:46), I never ran any faster. Performance disappointments aside I hope it has shown runners:

- They can be consistent (no matter how injury prone)
- Even with average talent like mine, as little as 30 – 40 miles repeated consistently can deliver impressive performance improvements. If you are injury prone and talented, you may far exceed my achievements using a similar approach.

Afterword

15th of August 2019

The pursuit of pleasure at the expense of pain, known as hedonism, is often considered the philosophy of the reckless. Live for today at the expense of tomorrow. The trouble is that tomorrow usually comes and the pursuit must begin again or the pain returns. If you've already conjured up images of alcohol, drugs, parties or Netflix binges, let me introduce you to the hedonism that was my Saturday morning. I wasn't falling out of a night-club, more bounding home from run training. Normally by this time (11am), I'd have run 16 kilometres with at least 10 of those at high intensity. Endorphins would be pulsating through my veins while I prepared a well-earned breakfast. Who knew that intense exercise could be *hedonistic* and that breakfast had to be *earned*? The tattoo on the back of my right calf translates as '*in the pursuit of excellence*', Saturday mornings were *in the pursuit of hedonism*.

Peeling the Layers of an Onion or Letting Go of the Armour

I ceased competitive running at the end of November last year. I continued to train almost as normal until March, partly because I wasn't sure what else to do. By then, I was hoping to have found a new goal or more accurately, the motivation to pursue one (such as a marathon). During the same period, I met a woman. She was a good runner. A combination of not wanting to let go of a former lover (running) and the excitement of a romance meant I continued to mix running and romance during this period. In reality, I was using this combination to put off dealing with myself and confronting the pain associated with developing a new identity (preferably one based around me!). The romance came to an end and the motivation to continue to run never came. It was as though my body knew that my mind was ready to move on and so it began to shut down. I was walking around as though there was a clamp attached to both of my achilles – running was no longer an option.

I've become a self-help junkie in the past year (prepare for a series of clichés that it turns out are actually true) and although I wasn't feeling great about life, I saw it as an opportunity for growth. In many respects, it was 10 years of failure and pain that eventually saw me flourish as an athlete. I would remind myself of this in the choppy waters ahead.

For most of the last 10 years, I've always had a crutch that has enabled me to avoid confronting myself. It has usually involved some combination of running and romance. In the absence of one or both, I have usually been able to find meaning in achievement (e.g. the pursuit of my PhD). It could be argued that this is simply part of the journey of growing up. This may be true in part but it is also a product of toxic perfectionism which has its roots in shame. [In understanding this and how to overcome it (we all have it to some extent), Brené Brown has become a hero of mine].

At 32, I decided I would finally throw away the crutches and have a go at just putting up with myself. It's described in the self-help world as akin to peeling away the layers of an onion. I can confirm it is very painful and just like the onion, it made me cry. Painful as it is, there is a certain satisfaction in the fact that I am no longer taking the painkillers (using external factors to maintain happiness). In other words, you feel the pain but as the pain subsides you know that's real too (ironically, learning to run and manage pain without painkillers is a smart strategy too). There were many things I didn't know about myself. Many of which are not pleasant. Confronting this was painful but eventually it has allowed me to become more compassionate toward myself and subsequently, others. [This blog originally started out as a blog on the superficial realities of life after running, but got deep and I ran with it].

Life after Running

The practicalities of not being a runner stretch far beyond running. For the guts of 17 years, the way I ate, slept, drank and planned my life sort of led back to when I was next running. Even during times I was not running, I was still a runner (i.e. living in the hope of one day returning). This time, I decided that no matter how good my legs felt, I would not run. Instead, I would try to adopt a healthy lifestyle of good food and daily exercise.

On an inter-personal level, I consciously tried to become less self-sufficient. Running is an individual sport and outside of sport, I am in a number of leadership roles (which I enjoy). I came to realise (with 11 months help from an extremely skilled counselor, thanks Richard!) that I had isolated myself emotionally by always being the runner or the leader. I have worked at expressing more vulnerability, clumsily at first, but I am gradually becoming more sophisticated and guess what, I have subsequently received more support [so simple, yet so difficult].

How does it work out?

I would love to say it's all perfectly wonderful now but it doesn't really work like that. I am no longer bathing in a sea of endorphins. Instead, I'm still in bed writing this whilst thinking I used to be fitter, have a more defined 6-pack etc. [I really need to finish this and hit the gym to appease that part of myself]. But equally, I'm not subject to the same roller-coaster of emotions that tend to happen when you are dependent on external factors. I have more time and freedom to socialise and explore other things (mainly myself at the moment). I try to pay attention to what excites me and follow that without trying to control the outcome.

I think that becoming aware of your limitations and mortality is important. It helps you pay attention to your passion whilst also trying to stay in the now. It has helped me to cultivate an appreciation for everything (& everyone) around me. It also helps to reduce time spent living a fear-based life. Fear is where the magic lies. In recent months, I have actively sought it out (e.g. playing full-contact rugby or doing a full somersault on a trampoline).

Where to from here?

The worst part of this process was being thrust into chaos initially. The chaos of being uncertain about who you are. It made me feel like a fraud and not knowing what parts of me were and were not real. To some extent, I needed to abandon some parts of me to see if they were real (e.g. the runner).

I am leaving the UK to take up a lecturing position back home in Ireland. I've got some broad areas (rather than definitive ends) I want to explore as they align with my interests and values.

The good news for readers of this blog is that I will finish the book *'Running from Injury. Why Do Runners Get Injured and How Do We Stop It?'*. My recent personal journey has helped me to see how much knowledge I gained in relation to running through the pain and suffering of injury. The next blog will be an outline of the book chapters, to put a little pressure on myself to crack on with it. I will also return to some running, as it will enhance the book. It is almost as though I need to get back to overcoming the limitations of my body (not as competitively) to finish the book in the best way I can.

Other things I'm excited about

Human Potential. I have interests in leadership, the broad ideals of higher education and male mental health, to mention a few. I want to write more, speak more and do more in relation to these topics alongside my work in science and running injury.

A note from the author

Thank you for reading this book. My mission with this book was to share ideas that might lead to more runners having fewer injuries. It is a personal project that I have self-funded both in terms of time and resources (including the cover, some illustrations and the associated marketing and social media). The only way that more runners will get to read this book is if they discover it. If you enjoyed this book, you could contribute to the mission by leaving a star rating and review on Amazon, that is how more runners will find it.

If you enjoyed this book but would like more specifics about the nuts and bolts of yoga, strength and conditioning, cross-training, the psychology of injury, specific training sessions and how to put it altogether you might like the complete catalogue of blogs (contents on the next page) that I have published in kindle and paperback version on amazon (**Tip:** if you are on a budget or cannot afford another book, you can google each individual title on the internet and read versions of them 1 by 1 for free).

Yours in running from injury,

Peter

The Complete Catalogue of Blogs

Available on amazon

Acknowledgements

To mum, for the dissatisfied curiosity, the desire to help others and a stubborn resilience.

To dad, for the ferocious self-discipline and the ability to apply myself to creatively solve any problem I choose.

To Gerry, for the gift of running, for the tenacity, enthusiasm, and passion to live my life to its fullest and for the example of what it means to be a good man, not just a good runner.

To my brother John, for being one half of my favourite two-man team.

To friends like Barry, Tim, Tom and many more, for reading my work, listening to my podcasts, attending my talks and boasting about me to others in the same way I boast about you to everyone else. I believe this is called unconditional man love.

To my mentors, Gerry, John Stacey, Professor Phil Jakeman, Caroline Mac Manus, Toni Rossiter, Alan Swanton, Professor Mark Johnson, Professor Grant Schofield and many more, time and opportunity are the greatest gifts you can give to anyone.

To Aisling and Megan, Alex Ferguson once said 'if they are good enough, they are old enough'. You are certainly good enough. Thank you for all your help with media and marketing.

To Dominika, thank you for this illustration and many others, but mostly for the patience required to get what is in my head into your pencil.

178

To my editor Cathal, life is funny. I remember running against you as teenagers on the rare occasions that neither of us were injured. You didn't really puncture my consciousness however, until you began to write. Reading your article '*Nil Desperandum*', while coaching at your parent club Emerald AC, was the first time I had ever seen someone capture the experience of being injured so perfectly. I became a fan and a follower of your journalism from that point onwards. Your writing has always inspired me to want to improve my own. You probably didn't realise the honour it was for me to meet you in a Dublin café in the autumn of 2017 and have you agree to being the editor of this book. The fact that you too had suffered injury and that you came from my 2nd home, Limerick, made it seem like faith to me. Thank you for questioning my reasoning and pushing me to make this better.

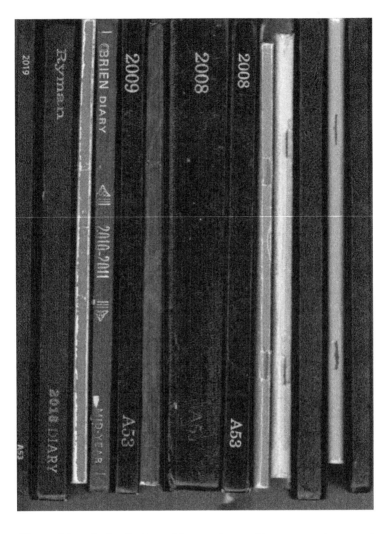

The training diaries that would go on to provide an accurate record for this book.

November 2004

Resume: Normal Programme

MONDAY 1 — SUBJECT: RSC @ 7pm — HOMEWORK — Date Due — Time Taken

- 2 laps warm up
- 3 mile @ 6.42 min pace
- 10 x 100 m
- 3 lap cool down
  = 10 miles.

TUESDAY 2 — SUBJECT: My house @ 4.20 pm — HOMEWORK — Date Due — Time Taken

- around Block
- up to GAA Pitch - 3 laps
- Back down
  = 10 miles @ 6.33 min pace
  = 1 hr 05 min 26 secs

WEDNESDAY 3 — SUBJECT: RSC - ATT @ 7pm — HOMEWORK — Date Due — Time Taken

- 3 laps
- 2 mile up (day to pick) P1 16
- 6 laps tempo : 21.05 (3.30 mn/km)
- 2 mile cool down
- 3 laps warm down
  = 10 miles

Week Total : 77 miles

THURSDAY 4 — SUBJECT: Long Run @ RSC 6pm — HOMEWORK — Date Due — Time Taken

- Ron in from house = 6 miles — 40 min
- over Ferrybank = 11 miles / 1hr 16 min
  = 17 miles

(Tired)
(Fucked)

FRIDAY 5 — SUBJECT: EASY DAY — HOMEWORK — Date Due — Time Taken

Around My house after school
@ 12.30 am

= easy

Comment: not Feeling to Gd

SATURDAY 6 — Clover @ 11am — HOMEWORK — Date Due — Time Taken
(Tough session)

- 2 k warm up
- 3, 4, 3.2, 3.2, 12.1, 1.14, 2, 2.3, 3, 3.2
- 12 k ladder session in top field
- 1 k warm down
  Total Session : 15 k TOTAL: 13 miles

SUNDAY 7 (Tired)

PotHaw @ 6pm + Evening 4 miles
@ 10am
- 13 miles
- up & reverse
- 1hr 30 min
(Feeling: reasonable)

The infamous 77-mile training week in 2004 (aged-17 years).

181

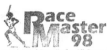

Provisional Results for All Competitors in finish order.

Place	Time	Name	Team	Race Age Category	Pace min/mile	Race No	Race Place
1	0:26:33	DUGGAN, Peter	St Josephs A.C	Men	05:18.5	62	1
2	0:26:40	LANGFORD, Mark	West Waterford A.C	Men	05:19.9	166	2
3	0:27:05	LEDINGHAM, James	West Waterford A.C	Men	05:24.9	57	3
4	0:27:09	O'SULLIVAN, Pat	Clonmel AC	Men	05:25.7	134	4
5	0:27:15	CUMMINS, Damien	St Josephs A.C	Men	05:26.9	73	5
6	0:27:31	HEFFERNAN, Pat	Fethard	Men	05:30.1	195	6
7	0:27:34	CURTIN, Noel	Youghal A.C	Men	05:30.7	121	7
8	0:27:44	STEPHENSON, Paul	Ferrybank	Men	05:32.7	124	8
9	0:28:00	FRANCIS, Peter	Ferrybank	Men	05:35.9	58	9
10	0:28:02	LACEY, Larry	St Josephs A.C	Men	05:36.3	64	10
11	0:28:19	BRUNNOCK, Johnny	Clonmel AC	Men	05:39.7	56	11
12	0:28:22	STILLWELL, Sean		Men	05:40.3	15	12
13	0:28:31	DUGGAN, Jack	St Josephs A.C	Men	05:42.1	47	13
14	0:28:34	MASON, Trevor	West Waterford A.C	Men	05:42.7	69	14
15	0:28:49	O'CONNOR, Johnny	West Waterford A.C	Men	05:45.7	127	15
16	0:29:11	LEARY, Andrew	West Waterford A.C	Men	05:50.1	175	16
17	0:29:24	O'LOUGHLIN, Michael	West Waterford A.C	Men	05:52.7	173	17
18	0:29:29	KELLY, Joe	West Waterford A.C	Men	05:53.7	217	18
19	0:29:38	MCCARTHY, Martin	West Waterford A.C	Men	05:55.5	55	19
20	0:29:40	CUMMINS, Sinead	St Josephs A.C	Ladies	05:55.9	65	20
21	0:29:47	DUNFORD, Michael	Sil cuilainn	Men	05:57.3	54	21
22	0:29:50	O'CONNER, Gearoid	Rathfarnham	Men	05:57.9	43	22
23	0:30:04	CARTHY, Jake	Kilmore A.C	Ladies	06:00.7	40	23
24	0:30:05	CANTWELL, Gerry	West Waterford A.C	Men	06:00.9	84	24
25	0:30:05	TRAVERS, Jason	West Waterford A.C	Men	06:00.9	85	25

The Ardmore 5-mile road race that would go on to become my reference point after I ran 26:48 in 2005.

Place	Boys Under 19	3000 Metres	Standard
1	Rory Chesser	Ennis Track	9.52.05
2	Cathal Dennehy	Emerald	9.08.96
3	Peter Francis	Ferrybank	9.24.93

I didn't realise in 2005, that my track competitor would eventually become the editor of this book. I also didn't know just how many injuries we both would suffer.

Table 1: Body composition data for an endurance athlete between 2008 – 2015.

Time Point	Body Mass (kg)	Lean Tissue Mass (kg)	Body Fat Mass (kg)	Body Fat (%)
10/11/2008	80.7	66.1	11.1	13.7
30/06/2010	85.0	65.9	15.4	18.1
28/10/2010	86.2	71.0	10.0	12.5
Between Intervention Summary (Mean of n= 12 DXA scans)				
2011 – 2014				
22/07/14	87.5	70.6	13.2	15.1
15/08/13	89.3	71.6	13.9	15.6
22/04/13	88.4	70.2	14.4	16.3
27/02/13	90.0	71.5	14.8	16.4
21/12/12	88.9	70.6	14.6	16.5
09/11/12	89.7	69.8	16.2	18.0
24/07/12	90.0	69.9	16.3	18.1
12/12/11	87.5	70.1	13.6	15.6
21/10/11	91.4	72.0	15.6	17.1
22/06/11	87.4	71.9	11.8	13.5
26/04/11	86.4	72.1	10.6	12.2
10/02/11	86.2	71.9	10.5	12.2
Average ± STDEV	88.6 ± 1.6	71.0 ± 0.9	13.8 ± 2.0	15.6 ± 2.0
Intervention 2				
03/04/2015	90.6	70.4	16.5	18.2
18/06/2015	86.2	71.2	11.2	13.0

The body beautiful: *When I was dependent solely on running for my athletic pursuits my body fat percentage and lean mass fluctuated according to when I was injured. I am leanest during brief breakthrough periods in 2008-2009 and 2010-2011 and when training for a triathlon in 2015.*

183

27 Monday
- 60 min
- CT easy

28 Tuesday
- 9 miles (Weights)
- 5 x 800m 60 sec rest (14:09)
- 5:18:00 m 90sec rest
- Set 1: 2:43, 2:40, 2:40, 2:40, 2:35
- Set 2: 2:32, 2:44, 2:33, 2:46
- 2:30

29 Wednesday
- 60 min
- Yoga

Thursday 30
- 8 x 400m in 80 sec (weights)
- 3 miles @ 5:47
- 8.6 miles

Friday 1
- 60 min CT
- easy

Saturday 2
- 6 miles
- 5 km
- Park Run
- 16:53

Sunday 3
- 8:45, 8:46, 7:46, 7:24, 7:14
- 7:21, 7:13, 7:25, 6:58, 7:23
- 10 mile

Total miles (49)

The 2nd attempt: Training was very different in my 2nd coming as a runner

	A	B	C	D	E	F	G	H	I
1		**Monday**	**Tuesday**	**Wednesday**	**Thursday**	**Friday**	**Saturday**	**Sunday**	**Total**
2	August 27th	4	11	weights	8	bike	8	12	39
3		circuits	tempo			2.5h	tempo		
4									
5	September 3rd	0	8.6	7.6	bike	Weights	10.6	13	40
6			Track	easy	2.5h				
7			Weights	Barefoot					
8	Sept 10th	weights	9.3	7.6	weights	10	14	0	41
9			Track			tempo			
10									
11	Sept 17th	weights	8.3	bike	8.3	weights	9.3	15	41
12				2-hrs			tempo		
13									
14	Sept 24th	weights	9.8	weights	8	rest	9.7	15	43
15			Track				tempo		
16									
17	Oct 1st	weights	8.7	bike	8	weights	8.8	15	41
18			Track	2-hrs					
19									
20	Oct 8th	weights	9.5	bike	8	weights	8.3	15	41
21			Track	2-hrs					
22									

2016 | 2016-2017 | Feb-July 2017 (NZ) | 2017-2018 | **2018-2019** | Limerick 2019 | Consistency | ⊕

Becoming a master of consistency: *the idea that I would ever have 3-years of consistent training data in an excel file, for a long time would have seemed like madness. In the end, I prided myself on my consistency and keeping a careful audit of same.*

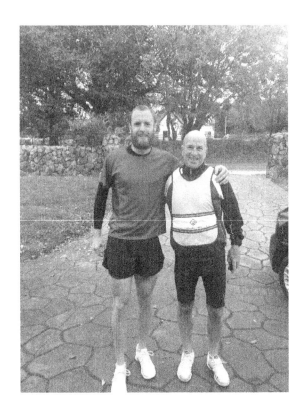

Meet the mentor: *October 2018, prior to a 15-mile run on the roads of my native Waterford. Gerry accompanied me on the bike for what would be my last long run before retirement. It was fitting the man who saw me into the sport 16-years earlier, guided me out the other side.*

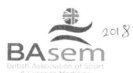

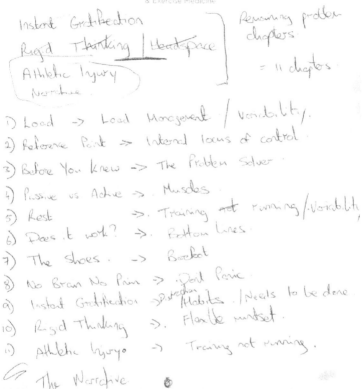

Instant Gratification

Rigid Thinking | Headspace

Athletic Injury

Narrative

Remaining problem chapters

= 11 chapters.

1) Load → Load Management / Variability.
2) Reference Point → Internal locus of control.
3) Before You Knew → The Problem Solver.
4) Passive vs Active → Muscles
5) Rest → Training not running / Variability
6) Does it work? → Bottom Lines.
7) The shoes. → Barefoot
8) No Brain No Pain → Don't Panic
9) Instant Gratification → Habits. / Needs to be done
10) Rigid Thinking → Flexible mindset.
11) Athletic Injury → Training not running.

↳ The Narrative

Doing some rough work for the book. Trying to get clear on what the problems were and what their opposites would look like.

187

References

1.	Dean HJ, Sellers EA. Children have type 2 diabetes too: an historical perspective. *Biochemistry and cell biology = Biochimie et biologie cellulaire.* 2015;93(5):425-429.

2.	Lieberman DE. The Story of the Human Body: Evolution, Health and Disease. *Family medicine.* 2016;48(10):822-823.

3.	Koopman JJ, van Bodegom D, Ziem JB, Westendorp RG. An Emerging Epidemic of Noncommunicable Diseases in Developing Populations Due to a Triple Evolutionary Mismatch. *The American journal of tropical medicine and hygiene.* 2016;94(6):1189-1192.

4.	Brown JP, Josse RG. 2002 clinical practice guidelines for the diagnosis and management of osteoporosis in Canada. *CMAJ : Canadian Medical Association journal = journal de l'Association medicale canadienne.* 2002;167(10 Suppl):S1-34.

5.	Francis P, Schofield G. From barefoot hunter gathering to shod pavement pounding. Where to from here? A narrative review. *BMJ open sport & exercise medicine.* 2020;6(1):e000577.

6.	Lysholm J, Wiklander J. Injuries in runners. *The American journal of sports medicine.* 1987;15(2):168-171.

7.	Fernandes HM. Physical activity levels in Portuguese adolescents: A 10-year trend analysis (2006-2016). *Journal of science and medicine in sport.* 2018;21(2):185-189.

8.	Kahneman D. *Thinking, fast and slow.* Macmillan; 2011.

9.   Gabbett TJ. The training-injury prevention paradox: should athletes be training smarter and harder? *British journal of sports medicine.* 2016;50(5):273-280.

10.   Hamstra-Wright KL, Coumbe-Lilley JE, Kim H, McFarland JA, Huxel Bliven KC. The influence of training and mental skills preparation on injury incidence and performance in marathon runners. *Journal of strength and conditioning research.* 2013;27(10):2828-2835.

11.   Hespanhol Junior LC, Pena Costa LO, Lopes AD. Previous injuries and some training characteristics predict running-related injuries in recreational runners: a prospective cohort study. *Journal of physiotherapy.* 2013;59(4):263-269.

12.   van Poppel D, de Koning J, Verhagen AP, Scholten-Peeters GG. Risk factors for lower extremity injuries among half marathon and marathon runners of the Lage Landen Marathon Eindhoven 2012: A prospective cohort study in the Netherlands. *Scandinavian journal of medicine & science in sports.* 2016;26(2):226-234.

13.   Bovens AM, Janssen GM, Vermeer HG, Hoeberigs JH, Janssen MP, Verstappen FT. Occurrence of running injuries in adults following a supervised training program. *International journal of sports medicine.* 1989;10 Suppl 3:S186-190.

14.   van Gent RN, Siem D, van Middelkoop M, van Os AG, Bierma-Zeinstra SM, Koes BW. Incidence and determinants of lower extremity running injuries in long distance runners: a systematic review. *British journal of sports medicine.* 2007;41(8):469-480; discussion 480.

15. Parker DT, Weitzenberg TW, Amey AL, Nied RJ. Group training programs and self-reported injury risk in female marathoners. *Clin J Sport Med.* 2011;21(6):499-507.

16. Bishop DJ, Granata C, Eynon N. Can we optimise the exercise training prescription to maximise improvements in mitochondria function and content? *Biochim Biophys Acta.* 2014;1840(4):1266-1275.

17. Ericsson KA. Training history, deliberate practice and elite sports performance: an analysis in response to Tucker and Collins review--what makes champions? In: *Br J Sports Med.* Vol 47. England2013:533-535.

18. Kornaat PR, Van de Velde SK. Bone marrow edema lesions in the professional runner. *Am J Sports Med.* 2014;42(5):1242-1246.

19. Stahl R, Luke A, Ma CB, et al. Prevalence of pathologic findings in asymptomatic knees of marathon runners before and after a competition in comparison with physically active subjects-a 3.0 T magnetic resonance imaging study. *Skeletal Radiol.* 2008;37(7):627-638.

20. Shaikh Z, Perry M, Morrissey D, Ahmad M, Del Buono A, Maffulli N. Achilles tendinopathy in club runners. *Int J Sports Med.* 2012;33(5):390-394.

21. Jelsing EJ, Finnoff J, Levy B, Smith J. The prevalence of fluid associated with the iliotibial band in asymptomatic recreational runners: an ultrasonographic study. *PM R.* 2013;5(7):563-567.

22. Finan PH, Buenaver LF, Bounds SC, et al. Discordance between pain and radiographic severity in knee osteoarthritis: findings from quantitative sensory

testing of central sensitization. *Arthritis Rheum.* 2013;65(2):363-372.

23. Hespanhol Junior LC, de Carvalho AC, Costa LO, Lopes AD. Lower limb alignment characteristics are not associated with running injuries in runners: Prospective cohort study. *Eur J Sport Sci.* 2016;16(8):1137-1144.

24. O'Sullivan P. It's time for change with the management of non-specific chronic low back pain. *British journal of sports medicine.* 2012;46(4):224-227.

25. Francis P, Whatman C, Sheerin K, Hume P, Johnson MI. The Proportion of Lower Limb Running Injuries by Gender, Anatomical Location and Specific Pathology: A Systematic Review. *Journal of sports science & medicine.* 2019;18(1):21-31.

26. Kovalak E, Atay T, Çetin C, Atay IM, Serbest MO. Is ACL reconstruction a prerequisite for the patients having recreational sporting activities? *Acta orthopaedica et traumatologica turcica.* 2018;52(1):37-43.

27. McAuliffe S, McCreesh K, Culloty F, Purtill H, O'Sullivan K. Can ultrasound imaging predict the development of Achilles and patellar tendinopathy? A systematic review and meta-analysis. *British journal of sports medicine.* 2016;50(24):1516-1523.

28. Taunton JE, Ryan MB, Clement DB, McKenzie DC, Lloyd-Smith DR, Zumbo BD. A retrospective case-control analysis of 2002 running injuries. *British journal of sports medicine.* 2002;36(2):95-101.

29. Lopes AD, Hespanhol Junior LC, Yeung SS, Costa LO. What are the main running-related musculoskeletal

injuries? A Systematic Review. *Sports Med.* 2012;42(10):891-905.

30.   Knobloch K, Yoon U, Vogt PM. Acute and overuse injuries correlated to hours of training in master running athletes. *Foot Ankle Int.* 2008;29(7):671-676.

31.   Puentedura EJ, Louw A. A neuroscience approach to managing athletes with low back pain. *Phys Ther Sport.* 2012;13(3):123-133.

32.   Rio E, Moseley L, Purdam C, et al. The pain of tendinopathy: physiological or pathophysiological? *Sports Med.* 2014;44(1):9-23.

33.   Francis P, Lyons M, Piasecki M, Mc Phee J, Hind K, Jakeman P. Measurement of muscle health in aging. *Biogerontology.* 2017;18(6):901-911.

34.   Lieberman D. *The story of the human body: evolution, health, and disease.* Vintage; 2014.

35.   Myer GD, Ford KR, Di Stasi SL, Foss KD, Micheli LJ, Hewett TE. High knee abduction moments are common risk factors for patellofemoral pain (PFP) and anterior cruciate ligament (ACL) injury in girls: is PFP itself a predictor for subsequent ACL injury? *Br J Sports Med.* 2015;49(2):118-122.

36.   Askling CM, Tengvar M, Saartok T, Thorstensson A. Acute first-time hamstring strains during high-speed running: a longitudinal study including clinical and magnetic resonance imaging findings. *Am J Sports Med.* 2007;35(2):197-206.

37.   Fitzharris N, Jones G, Jones A, Francis P. The first prospective injury audit of league of Ireland footballers. *BMJ Open Sport & Exercise Medicine.* 2017;In press.

38.   Demontis GC, Germani MM, Caiani EG, Barravecchia I, Passino C, Angeloni D. Human Pathophysiological

Adaptations to the Space Environment. *Frontiers in physiology.* 2017;8:547.

39. Ferrando AA, Stuart CA, Brunder DG, Hillman GR. Magnetic resonance imaging quantitation of changes in muscle volume during 7 days of strict bed rest. *Aviation, space, and environmental medicine.* 1995;66(10):976-981.

40. Bleakley CM, Glasgow P, MacAuley DC. PRICE needs updating, should we call the POLICE? *British journal of sports medicine.* 2012;46(4):220-221.

41. Lieberman DE. What we can learn about running from barefoot running: an evolutionary medical perspective. *Exercise and sport sciences reviews.* 2012;40(2):63-72.

42. Trinkaus E. Anatomical evidence for the antiquity of human footwear use. *Journal of Archaeological Science.* 2005;32(10):1515-1526.

43. Kuttruff JT, DeHart SG, O'Brien MJ. 7500 years of prehistoric footwear from arnold research cave, missouri. *Science.* 1998;281(5373):72-75.

44. Hoffmann P. Conclusions drawn from a comparative study of the feet of barefooted and shoe-wearing peoples. *Am J Orthop Surg.* 1905;2(2):105-136.

45. Davis IS. The re-emergence of the minimal running shoe. *The Journal of orthopaedic and sports physical therapy.* 2014;44(10):775-784.

46. Engle ET, Morton DJ. Notes on foot disorders among natives of the Belgian Congo. *JBJS.* 1931;13(2):311-318.

47. James C. Footprints and feet of natives of the Solomon Islands. *The Lancet.* 1939;234(6070):1390-1394.

48.   D'Août K, Pataky TC, De Clercq D, Aerts P. The effects of habitual footwear use: foot shape and function in native barefoot walkers. *Footwear Science.* 2009;1(2):81-94.

49.   Rao UB, Joseph B. The influence of footwear on the prevalence of flat foot. A survey of 2300 children. *The Journal of bone and joint surgery British volume.* 1992;74(4):525-527.

50.   Devereaux MD, Lachmann SM. Athletes attending a sports injury clinic--a review. *British journal of sports medicine.* 1983;17(4):137-142.

51.   Barrow GW, Saha S. Menstrual irregularity and stress fractures in collegiate female distance runners. *The American journal of sports medicine.* 1988;16(3):209-216.

52.   Jakobsen BW, Kroner K, Schmidt SA, Kjeldsen A. Prevention of injuries in long-distance runners. *Knee surgery, sports traumatology, arthroscopy : official journal of the ESSKA.* 1994;2(4):245-249.

53.   Ryan MB, Valiant GA, McDonald K, Taunton JE. The effect of three different levels of footwear stability on pain outcomes in women runners: a randomised control trial. *Br J Sports Med.* 2011;45(9):715-721.

54.   Knapik JJ, Trone DW, Swedler DI, et al. Injury reduction effectiveness of assigning running shoes based on plantar shape in Marine Corps basic training. *Am J Sports Med.* 2010;38(9):1759-1767.

55.   Knapik JJ, Trone DW, Tchandja J, Jones BH. Injury-reduction effectiveness of prescribing running shoes on the basis of foot arch height: summary of military investigations. *J Orthop Sports Phys Ther.* 2014;44(10):805-812.

56.   Echarri JJ, Forriol F. The development in footprint morphology in 1851 Congolese children from urban and rural areas, and the relationship between this and wearing shoes. *Journal of pediatric orthopedics Part B.* 2003;12(2):141-146.

57.   Holowka NB, Wallace IJ, Lieberman DE. Foot strength and stiffness are related to footwear use in a comparison of minimally- vs. conventionally-shod populations. *Scientific reports.* 2018;8(1):3679.

58.   Franklin S, Grey MJ, Heneghan N, Bowen L, Li FX. Barefoot vs common footwear: A systematic review of the kinematic, kinetic and muscle activity differences during walking. *Gait & posture.* 2015;42(3):230-239.

59.   Robbins SE, Gouw GJ, Hanna AM. Running-related injury prevention through innate impact-moderating behavior. *Medicine and science in sports and exercise.* 1989;21(2):130-139.

60.   Stolwijk NM, Duysens J, Louwerens JW, van de Ven YH, Keijsers NL. Flat feet, happy feet? Comparison of the dynamic plantar pressure distribution and static medial foot geometry between Malawian and Dutch adults. *PloS one.* 2013;8(2):e57209.

61.   Altman AR, Davis IS. Prospective comparison of running injuries between shod and barefoot runners. *Br J Sports Med.* 2016;50(8):476-480.

62.   Willems TM, Ley C, Goetghebeur E, Theisen D, Malisoux L. Motion-Control Shoes Reduce the Risk of Pronation-Related Pathologies in Recreational Runners: A Secondary Analysis of a Randomized Controlled Trial. *The Journal of orthopaedic and sports physical therapy.* 2021;51(3):135-143.

63. Barnes KR, Kilding AE. A Randomized Crossover Study Investigating the Running Economy of Highly-Trained Male and Female Distance Runners in Marathon Racing Shoes versus Track Spikes. *Sports medicine (Auckland, NZ).* 2019;49(2):331-342.

64. Muniz-Pardos B, Sutehall S, Angeloudis K, Guppy FM, Bosch A, Pitsiladis Y. Recent Improvements in Marathon Run Times Are Likely Technological, Not Physiological. *Sports Medicine.* 2021;51(3):371-378.

65. Sichting F, Holowka NB, Hansen OB, Lieberman DE. Effect of the upward curvature of toe springs on walking biomechanics in humans. *Scientific reports.* 2020;10(1):14643.

66. Johnson CD, Tenforde AS, Outerleys J, Reilly J, Davis IS. Impact-Related Ground Reaction Forces Are More Strongly Associated With Some Running Injuries Than Others. *The American journal of sports medicine.* 2020;48(12):3072-3080.

67. O'Sullivan P. It's time for change with the management of non-specific chronic low back pain. In: *Br J Sports Med.* Vol 46. England2012:224-227.

68. Nielsen RO, Ronnow L, Rasmussen S, Lind M. A prospective study on time to recovery in 254 injured novice runners. *PloS one.* 2014;9(6):e99877.

69. Francis P, Thornley I, Jones A, Johnson MI. Pain and Function in the Runner a Ten (din) uous Link. *Medicina (Kaunas, Lithuania).* 2020;56(1).

70. Kahneman D. *Thinking, fast and slow.* London: Penguin; 2012.

71. Mischel Wa. *The marshmallow test : understanding self-control and how to master it.*

72. Kübler-Ross E, Wessler S, Avioli LVJJ. On death and dying. 1972;221(2):174-179.

73.   Willwacher S, Fischer KM, Rohr E, Trudeau MB, Hamill J, Brüggemann GP. Surface Stiffness and Footwear Affect the Loading Stimulus for Lower Extremity Muscles When Running. *Journal of strength and conditioning research.* 2020.

74.   Lum D, Tan F, Pang J, Barbosa TM. Effects of intermittent sprint and plyometric training on endurance running performance. *Journal of sport and health science.* 2019;8(5):471-477.

75.   Chong CS, Tsunaka M, Tsang HW, Chan EP, Cheung WM. Effects of yoga on stress management in healthy adults: A systematic review. *Alternative therapies in health and medicine.* 2011;17(1):32-38.

76.   Little JP, Safdar A, Wilkin GP, Tarnopolsky MA, Gibala MJ. A practical model of low-volume high-intensity interval training induces mitochondrial biogenesis in human skeletal muscle: potential mechanisms. *The Journal of physiology.* 2010;588(Pt 6):1011-1022.

77.   Dekker JM, Crow RS, Folsom AR, et al. Low heart rate variability in a 2-minute rhythm strip predicts risk of coronary heart disease and mortality from several causes: the ARIC Study. Atherosclerosis Risk In Communities. *Circulation.* 2000;102(11):1239-1244.

78.   Aguiar-Oliveira MH, Bartke A. Growth Hormone Deficiency: Health and Longevity. *Endocrine reviews.* 2019;40(2):575-601.

79.   Nutt DJ, Lingford-Hughes A, Erritzoe D, Stokes PR. The dopamine theory of addiction: 40 years of highs and lows. *Nature reviews Neuroscience.* 2015;16(5):305-312.

80.   Ozgok Kangal MK, Regan JP. Wound Healing. In: *StatPearls.* Treasure Island (FL): StatPearls Publishing

81.   Cresci GA, Bawden E. Gut Microbiome: What We Do and Don't Know. *Nutrition in clinical practice : official publication of the American Society for Parenteral and Enteral Nutrition.* 2015;30(6):734-746.

82.   Frankl VE. *Man's search for meaning.* Simon and Schuster; 1985.

83.   Peters S. *The chimp paradox: The mind management program to help you achieve success, confidence, and happiness.* TarcherPerigee; 2013.

84.   Bowser BJ, Rose WC, McGrath R, Salerno J, Wallace J, Davis IS. Effect of Footwear on Dynamic Stability during Single-leg Jump Landings. *International journal of sports medicine.* 2017;38(6):481-486.

85.   Ridge ST, Olsen MT, Bruening DA, et al. Walking in Minimalist Shoes Is Effective for Strengthening Foot Muscles. *Medicine and science in sports and exercise.* 2019;51(1):104-113.

86.   Cudejko T, Gardiner J, Akpan A, D'Août K. Minimal shoes improve stability and mobility in persons with a history of falls. *Scientific reports.* 2020;10(1):21755.

87.   Mizushima J, Keogh JWL, Maeda K, et al. Long-term effects of school barefoot running program on sprinting biomechanics in children: A case-control study. *Gait & posture.* 2021;83:9-14.